Praise for the Book

"Dan Morhaim's message is a must-read for anyone who is facing end-of-life crisis issues and concerns, whether it be for themselves or for a family member or loved one. When so many others shun the topic, Dan Morhaim addresses the situation with clarity, insight, and sensitivity."—**Montel Williams**

"Dan Morhaim provides key insights into ways to navigate the difficult end-of-life journey traveled by individuals and families across the country. This valuable guide offers thoughtful policy analysis while also highlighting essential considerations for you and your loved ones so that you can make decisions consistent with your values and wishes."—**Chris Van Hollen**, US Senator

"I applaud the Morhaims' commitment to humanity as they encourage us to embrace the reality of our mortality. This book demonstrates that we have power to control our destiny, including the transition to death. We are best served by doing so, for ourselves and for those we inevitably leave behind."—**David O. Fakunle**, Cofounder/CEO, DiscoverME/RecoverME: Enrichment through the African Oral Tradition/Associate Faculty, Johns Hopkins Bloomberg School of Public Health

"End-of-life care is increasingly complex and deserves informed, clear decision making. This invaluable book gives practical, wise, and deeply compassionate support as we traverse the final days of our human journey."—**Tara Brach**, author of *Radical Acceptance: Embracing Your Life with the Heart of a Buddha*

"Dr. Morhaim's excellent book provides practical advice for navigating the medical, emotional, social, and spiritual complexities of the serious illness journey. It does so in a way that promotes patient-centered decision-making, especially at life's end, protecting patient and family alike. It's a clearly written and much-needed guide that all can use."—**Robert L. Fine**, MD, FACP, FAAHPM, Clinical Director, Baylor Scott & White Health, Office of Clinical Ethics and Palliative Care

"Dr. Morhaim's *Preparing for a Better End* is both approachable and comprehensive for providers and patients alike. This roadmap for end-of-life care and decision-making explores many different scenarios while helping to demystify this deeply personal experience that each of us must navigate."—**Robert Barish**, MD, MBA, Vice Chancellor for Health Affairs, University of Illinois at Chicago/Professor of Emergency Medicine, University of Illinois College of Medicine

"Bringing the individual and the family into health care decision making has to be one of medicine's core values. This book keeps that as its focus, while providing sound, practical advice about navigating the health care system when things get tough. In that way, Dr. Morhaim helps patients, families, providers, and society. I recommend this book highly."—**Angelo Volandes**, MD, Cofounder/President, Advance Care Planning Decisions/Associate Professor of Medicine, Harvard Medical School/Massachusetts General Hospital, author of *The Conversation: A Revolutionary Plan for End-of-Life Care*

"While we prepare for several milestones in life such as marriage, children, or even retirement, too often we as a society overlook the importance of advance care planning. Dan Morhaim's *Preparing for a Better End* provides the framework, expectations, and guidance needed to navigate this intimidating process and helps to break it down in a digestible manner that gives everyone the confidence needed to plan for the best end-of-life experience possible."—**Elizabeth Clayborne**, MD, MA in Bioethics, Emergency Medicine Physician, University of Maryland Department of Emergency Medicine

"*Preparing for a Better End* is a powerful, persuasive, very readable book on the importance of considering and planning for our eventual deaths. I am looking forward to using this exceptionally compassionate, honest, and forthright book in my ongoing practice and sharing it with the entire palliative team."—**Evangeline Calland**, Hospital Chaplain, Sentara Martha Jefferson Hospital

"Sometimes the simplest innovations are the hardest. In this case, it's completing advance directives. Dr. Morhaim makes a compelling case why this is something we should all do, and he shares how our digital age makes it easy and accessible." —**Molly Coye**, MD, MPH, Executive-in-Residence, AVIA Health

"*Preparing for a Better End* unfolds like a leisurely walk with a mentor. You find yourself understanding things that others have tried to tell you for years. Morhaim uses an array of stories from a lifetime of diverse experience to teach, not preach. Advance care planning is not new, but this is a fresh guide for why and how to use it."—**Nathan Kottkamp**, Founder/Chair, National Healthcare Decisions Day

"Prevention and planning are the best ways to manage complex health care issues. This book gives the reader both the reasons and methods to do so, the 'why' and the 'how to,' especially when facing serious illness. It's about empowerment and respect for individual values, something we can all use in difficult situations." —**Clarence Lam**, MD, MPH, Director, Preventive Medicine Residency Program/ Assistant Scientist, Johns Hopkins Bloomberg School of Public Health

"*Preparing for a Better End* is an excellent resource for anyone working through the process of making decisions about end-of-life care. It is suitable for a broad range of people, including people who have different convictions about certain end-of-life questions. I heartily recommend Dr. Morhaim's work to other clergy and religious leaders."—**Rev. Jason A. Poling**, DMin, Episcopal Priest/Director, Doctor of Ministry Program, St. Mary's Seminary & University

Preparing
for a
Better End

EXPERT LESSONS ON DEATH AND DYING

FOR YOU AND YOUR LOVED ONES

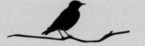

Dan Morhaim, MD

With Shelley Morhaim

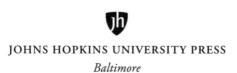

JOHNS HOPKINS UNIVERSITY PRESS

Baltimore

Note to the Reader: This book is not meant to substitute for medical care and treatment should not be based solely on its contents. Instead, treatment must be developed in a dialogue between the individual and his or her physician. This book has been written to help with that dialogue.

Johns Hopkins University Press
2715 North Charles Street
Baltimore, Maryland 21218-4363
www.press.jhu.edu

Library of Congress Cataloging-in-Publication Data

Names: Morhaim, Dan, author. | Morhaim, Shelley, 1949– author.
Title: Preparing for a better end : expert lessons on death and dying for you
    and your loved ones / Dan Morhaim, MD, with Shelley Morhaim.
Description: Baltimore : Johns Hopkins University Press, 2020. |
    Includes index.
Identifiers: LCCN 2019059955 | ISBN 9781421439167 (hardcover) |
    ISBN 9781421439174 (paperback) | ISBN 9781421439181 (ebook)
Subjects: LCSH: Right to die—Popular works. | Terminal care—
    Popular works. | Death—Planning—Popular works.
Classification: LCC R726 .M6923 2020 | DDC 179.7—dc23
LC record available at https://lccn.loc.gov/2019059955

A catalog record for this book is available from the British Library.

Special discounts are available for bulk purchases of this book. For more information, please contact Special Sales at specialsales@press.jhu.edu.

Johns Hopkins University Press uses environmentally friendly book materials, including recycled text paper that is composed of at least 30 percent post-consumer waste, whenever possible.

For Helen and Maude, our newest teachers
And in memory of our parents and grandparents

Contents

PREPARING FOR A BETTER END

Why Not the Best of Both Worlds?

———

Life is pleasant. Death is peaceful. It's the transition that's troublesome.
—Isaac Asimov

To the well-organized mind, death is but the next great adventure.
—J. K. Rowling

The previous book I wrote with my wife, *The Better End: Surviving (and Dying) on Your Own Terms in Today's Modern Medical World*, examined our unique situation as the first generation in human history to have a meaningful say in how we will experience the dying process.

When I was asked to write again on the topic, I began to look at how much had changed in the intervening 10 years. Issues that were formerly marginal had now moved to the center of medical-legal-political discussion. Treatments and options for care had multiplied and evolved. In preparing for a better end, we now have more that we must take into account.

We live in an era of medical marvels. In the United States, life expectancy has increased by some 30 years from what it was a century ago. New treatments for debilitating and life-threatening diseases are being developed every year. Yet despite the superb medical care available in the United States, our death rate remains the same as the poorest nation on earth: one per person.

We don't know the time or the manner, but we know that one day death will come for us. That is our common human destiny. But we are different from all the generations that preceded us in

1

one important respect: we can influence how that destiny unfolds. That gives us new responsibility and also new power. Let's take advantage of that.

We know this topic is scary and that it's one we would prefer not to think or talk about. But if you follow the steps outlined here, you'll be more in control and more prepared to face whatever comes. This will give you the confidence to ask questions and get the answers you deserve. The payoff is hope and comfort for you and your family.

To put this into perspective, let's time-travel back 100 years . . .

At age 50, Harold Johnson, a farmer in western Pennsylvania, had already exceeded the average life expectancy for his time. Two of his siblings and one of his own children had passed away before reaching the age of 20. A daughter-in-law had died in childbirth. But Harold had enjoyed a full life with Martha, his wife of 26 years, with whom he had four living children and two grandchildren.

But now Harold's life was nearing its close. It had started the past winter when a bad cold had lingered. It seemed to accelerate the pains he occasionally felt in his chest after physical labor, and he had to ask his family to manage the spring planting without his help. As summer wore on, even the least exertion left him short of breath. Finally, he lacked the strength to get out of bed most days.

Dr. Reed, the Johnson family physician, had trained at the University of Pennsylvania Medical College in Philadelphia and kept up with all the latest advances. He'd managed to buy Harold a few years of pain relief using nitroglycerin tablets, but as Harold's heart muscle deteriorated, his blood flow decreased. His color became pale, and fluid began to build up in his lungs, making his breathing even harder. Finally, pneumonia set in.

The doctor was called and confirmed what Harold and Martha suspected: the end was drawing near. Dr. Reed's scientific medical bag was fairly empty. The antibiotics that could have cured Harold's pneumonia wouldn't be discovered for another decade. The cardiac surgery, appliances, and medications that could have repaired his heart's function were even more distantly removed—50 or more years in the future. But Dr. Reed wasn't entirely helpless. He'd known the Johnson family for years, and just his presence provided a degree of comfort and dignity to Harold's dying. Dr. Reed made daily house calls, checking Harold's pulse, charting the course of his fever and other symptoms, counseling Harold and Martha, and letting them know when it was time to summon the children and grandchildren, the minister from their church, and Harold's brother from Ohio.

Pneumonia used to be known as "the old man's friend" because it brought a relatively quick and painless end. As Harold's health failed, his family and friends came to say goodbye. They talked with Harold about his life, both the good times and the difficult ones.

As the days progressed, Harold's breathing became more labored, then shallower. He drifted in and out of consciousness. Finally, he lapsed into a coma. With Martha at his side, his children and grandchildren surrounding the bed, Harold breathed his last.

Now fast-forward 100 years . . .

At the age of 83, Harold's grandson Bill had already outlived his ancestor by 30-plus years. His own three children and five grandchildren all survived into adulthood, and he'd lived to welcome his first great-grandchild. Bill and his wife, Alice, lived an active lifestyle until Bill was diagnosed with prostate cancer at age 75. Surgery and chemotherapy kept the cancer in remission for a number of years, but eventually it returned and this time did not respond to treatment. As the cancer spread throughout his body, Bill followed the advice of his oncologist, radiologist, surgeon, and internist. While all of them were highly trained and well versed in the course of Bill's disease, none of them knew Bill or Alice well as individuals. When Bill's condition deteriorated beyond the help of surgery, his surgeon dropped out of the medical team. When chemotherapy and radiation were no longer options, those specialists also signed off of Bill's case. His internist prescribed painkillers and made sure the disease was tracked with all appropriate tests; but when Bill's condition grew even worse, he was moved into the hospital, where his care was largely managed by hospital-based physicians on rotation who were strangers to Bill and his family.

Bill underwent multiple hospitalizations over the last 18 months of his life. His children and grandchildren paid visits, but the machinery and organization of the modern medical establishment that kept Bill alive those extra months served also to erect a wall between him and his family.

The same type of pneumonia that took his grandfather brought on his final hospitalization. With modern antibiotics, the pneumonia was quickly defeated, leaving Bill's heart to give out when his liver stopped functioning. But instead of dying surrounded by loved ones at his home, he died alone in his ICU (intensive care unit) cubicle, surrounded by monitors, machines, and intravenous lines, his lungs inflated by a ventilator. Since no one on staff felt comfortable declaring the end to be imminent, Alice had gone home for the night, physically exhausted and emotionally drained by the hospital deathwatch.

WHY NOT THE BEST OF BOTH WORLDS?

It's not hard to see what's wrong and what's right in each of these scenarios. In the first one, Harold gets the benefit of personalized, humane care, with family and friends nearby, but he lacks the life-saving advantages of modern medicine. In the second one, thanks to medical advances, Bill enjoys a longer, healthier life, but in his final illness he exchanges the human touch for a succession of specialists, lab tests, X-rays, and hospitalizations. The whole person is reduced to a collection of failing organs and therapies, and he dies isolated from his family and community.

Why can't we have the best of both these worlds? We are the first generation in human history that can actively participate in not only our own health and well-being but also in our experience of death and dying. Of course, this won't be true for all of us. Some will die by a sudden lethal stroke or coronary blockage, some by accident or other trauma, but the overwhelming majority will succumb to illnesses that once were quickly fatal but are now treatable: cancer, heart ailments, kidney failure, and degenerative diseases. Thus, for most of us, while the exact moment of death is uncertain, generally we can begin to define its circumstances. I come to this topic both as a physician and as a state legislator, not to mention as a human who will one day experience my own last breath.

Today, when we face the end of our lives, we have a better sense of what is happening and why. We can approach death with a greater degree of consciousness and more information than any of the billions of humans who preceded us. This gives us unprecedented control of how, when, and where we die. Instead of being buffeted entirely by the forces of nature and the health care system, there is now some self-determination available to us in approaching our final days.

To some degree, this new encounter with the dying process mirrors changes in how we deal with that other universal human experience: childbirth. Once medical science had more to offer, childbirth underwent an evolution from attendance by midwives at home to high-tech hospital deliveries managed by trained obstetrical surgeons. Infants and mothers were saved who would have died in former times, but the experience became isolating for the mother and her family. The requirements of scientific control came to dominate the spiritual and emotional values of simple human connection and the joys of the birth experience. But over the last few decades, parents and some medical professionals have demanded changes that re-humanize the birth process without sacrificing any health benefits. We now see fathers and significant others included in the delivery room. Many hospitals provide homelike birthing centers and support for the laboring mother in the form of nurse-midwives, birth coaches, and prenatal classes for both parents. Independent birthing centers are available in some locations, and home births under careful supervision by midwives are coming back. And as it turns out, rethinking the birthing experience has led to even better health outcomes for mothers and babies. This evolution is still under way, but it began and continues because ordinary people demanded the "best of both worlds." Now as the baby boom generation reaches its senior years, as new lifesaving medical treatments are announced almost weekly, and as our health care system confronts a crisis of affordability, the need is urgent for ordinary people to demand participation in end-of-life decisions, to insist on having the best of both worlds.

A core American value is respect for individual rights. We cherish our autonomy and our ability to make personal choices about how we lead our lives. We raise objections when we perceive inappropriate incursions on our freedoms. Yet in the area of end-of-life care, we collectively fail to employ the means available to us and so abdicate an opportunity. It's puzzling that, in this one area, there's a disconnect between what we say we want and how we behave. What, then, will it take for us to move ourselves from inaction to action? In addition to exploring the many reasons to take action, this book will resonate, I hope, with this central American value. I hope that readers will recognize the power provided by an advance directive and end-of-life care planning and will take advantage of these valuable tools. Further, I hope that you, reader, will encourage others to do the same. Not only will you be doing the right thing for yourself; you will be doing the right thing for your family and community.

When I give talks on this subject, I always include the following 10-second exercise. I invite you to try it now. Just imagine that the end of your life is coming. Where are you exactly? Who is there with you? What's going on? What would you want in your last months, weeks, days, hours, and minutes of your life? What sort of care? What fits your personal worldview, life perspective, religion, and spiritual values?

I've asked those questions to thousands of people, and the answers are always the same: Almost everyone wants to be at home, with friends and family, and pain free. No one says they'd like to be killed in a fiery car crash or drown in a swimming accident or be left in an intensive care unit tied to machines and monitors, long past any hope of recovery, with family kept away down the hall.

The Stanford School of Medicine reported that 80% of Americans would prefer to die at home if possible.

According to the Stanford School of Medicine, studies have shown that approximately 80% of Americans would prefer to die at home if possible. Despite this, 60% of Americans die in acute care hospitals, 20% in nursing homes, and only 20% at home. Not every patient will want to die at home. Dying at home is not favored in certain cultures, and some patients may wish not to die at home out of concern that they might be a burden on their family.

My answer is the same as those of most Americans. I want to be at home, with family and friends around me. I want to be kept pain free and drift into whatever is next. What do you want?

These are deep questions, not easy to answer, but well worth pondering. In order to address them, we must begin with a consideration of our own ideas about and experiences with death.

This book is an attempt to set forth the possible choices that we and our loved ones may face in the course of the dying process. It examines both the medical and legal realities and also the options available for decision-making. While there is probably no more difficult topic to think about than one's own death, there is also the inescapable fact that each of us will die. By thinking about this now, we can know more confidently that our most deeply held values will be reflected in the choices made by us or for us at the end of life.

The middle of a health care crisis is the worst time to make difficult decisions, yet it is often exactly when we are called on to do so. The emotional impact of a medical crisis shouldn't be under-estimated. Serious illness—whether one's own or that of a spouse, close friend, or family member—is a recognized source of acute stress. During these times our judgment can become clouded, no matter how levelheaded or stoic we may normally be. Complex medical, financial, and spiritual issues demand attention, and they often must be resolved under severe time constraints. Conflicts can rise to the surface, and squabbles may break out between otherwise close and compatible family members. This is a poor time to be making important decisions, but it's precisely the moment when such decisions must be made. I've seen these episodes as a physician caring for patients and families, and I've also experienced them in my own life as a patient, friend, or family member. That is why I say it's better to have dealt in advance with as many difficult issues as possible.

Another stress factor is the current health care system in the United States. Most of us feel manipulated by its complex bureaucracy—with the rules, regulations, and directives coming from multiple sources, many of which may be unfamiliar to us. The intricacy (some would say the irrationality) of our system makes it difficult to navigate. At one state legislative hearing, I asked a roomful of health care experts to raise their hand if they could accurately estimate how much a hospital visit for a routine illness, like appendicitis, might cost and how much they'd have to pay out of pocket to the hospital, doctors, and pharmacy after insurance covered its share. No one could answer that question, a testament to the confusions in our system.

This is especially true when it comes to serious illness or injury. We trust and hope that the system will manage things and make us better, and it often does, even if later, when the paperwork hits, we are at a loss to understand what's going on.

Contemplating one's own death is hard. It can be like trying to look directly at the sun, but it can also be a way of helping us appreciate life more. The practice of planning ahead offers something rare and important in our modern medical system. It's an opportunity to exert influence. This empowerment in itself is often comforting. It's like being at sea in a small boat: you can't control the weather and waves, but it's good to have a rudder with which to guide your course.

I once thought of giving this book the subtitle "Take Control of the End of Your Life . . . Please," playing off the classic Henny Youngman joke. And it's true. When you take control of the end of your life, everyone is better off. The "Please" is my plea to patients (as doctors, we don't want to make these tough decisions for them) and to individuals (as legislators, we don't want to continually legislate these matters) and to my family and friends (because I care about them).

My goal is to put you in charge of your care in a way that matches your values and wishes. The end of life is more than a final diagnosis, more than a "cause of death" on a government certificate, more than legal forms or paperwork. Nowadays, it has become an exploration of circumstances and decisions that, previously, few people ever had the chance to consider.

It may seem difficult at first to tackle this project: getting the forms, thinking about them, engaging others, completing them, and storing them appropriately. But if you do, you will find yourself breathing a deep sigh of relief when it's over. You'll know that you've done the right thing according to your own personal beliefs, that you've spared others anguish and struggle, and that you've made decisions about the medical care you'll receive, decisions that will be honored. You'll be happy you did it.

While it's true that no one gets out of here alive, our ability to contemplate the dying process has profound implications. Like all journeys, it begins with small steps and attention to details. And it opens to us a grand vista of life with the breadth of the human experience.

THE SOLUTION: ADVANCE DIRECTIVES
TO MAKE OUR WISHES KNOWN

In 1991, the Self-Determination Act was passed by the US Congress and signed into law by President George H. W. Bush. The act specifies that individuals have the right to medical decision-making, including the right to accept or refuse treatment. The act permits individuals to create an advance directive to spell out these choices, and it requires that health care facilities provide information about advance directives when patients enter the system. Additionally, a facility cannot use the presence or absence of an advance directive to refuse care to a patient.

An advance directive is a straightforward way, legal in all 50 states, to designate end-of-life care decisions and make them work for you. Advance directives are official documents, and they are available at no cost or very little cost. Some are online, such as MyDirectives, Five Wishes, and CAKE. Advance directives can also be obtained from your attorney, hospital, or state government, most commonly through the state health department or the state attorney general's office. At the end of this book, the Resources section lists where you can find more information.

Some have voiced concerns that advance directives may not be honored by health care providers. This mostly occurs when providers are unfamiliar with their use. One way to ameliorate this situation is by making advance directives a normal part of every patient's medical record. As the medical world becomes more accustomed to the presence of advance directives, medical personnel will accept the legal and moral obligation to follow their provisions.

Advance directive forms are easy to fill out. They are clear, well organized, and only a few pages long. Their main cost is in time: taking the time to think about what sort of care you want should you ever be in a situation where you can't make medical decisions for yourself. You will want to talk about these choices with family and other advisors (doctors, clergy, lawyers), though this is not required. Fill out the form, file it in a safe but easily accessible place, give a copy to your health care provider and those who would be involved, and let a few trusted people know where it's kept. That's it.

WHAT IS AN ADVANCE DIRECTIVE?

Advance directives are also known as "living wills" or "medical power of attorney," but I will use the term "advance directive" throughout. Typically they consist of four parts:

1. Choosing the kind of care you want: This part is titled, variously, "Living Will," "Treatment Preferences," or "Instructions for Health Care." This part is where you specify details about your medical treatment and values.

2. Choosing someone to act on your behalf when you cannot: This section is titled "Medical Power of Attorney" or "Health Care Agent." If you become unable to make your own health care choices, the person or persons you name will have the authority to do it for you.

3. After-death instructions: This includes instructions about organ or body donation, disposition of the body, and funeral arrangements.

4. Documentation: This refers to the process of signing and witnessing the document that ensures your advance directive is legal and will be followed.

In the following chapters I discuss each of these elements in more detail. I also discuss the specifics of death and dying. One day I hope that completing an advance directive will become as accepted and normal a responsibility as maintaining a driver's license, paying your taxes, or saving money for your retirement. It's the right and responsible thing to do. As already noted, reading and thinking about such specifics can sometimes be difficult, but you will need this information to make an informed judgment about your personal choices.

This book was written before the COVID-19 pandemic began. Over the last few months, preparedness and the lack thereof have become front-burner issues for governments, the health care community, and the public. The tragedies faced by so many families have underscored the unpredictability of medical emergencies as well as the comfort that comes from thinking about difficult issues in advance whenever possible. We never know what's going to happen to any of us personally or to our family or friends. Now more than ever, advance care planning is essential.

My Dog Got Better Care
Than My Mother

A belief in hell and the knowledge that every ambition is doomed to frustration at the hands of a skeleton have never prevented the majority of human beings from behaving as though death were no more than an unfounded rumor.
—ALDOUS HUXLEY

THE BASICS: LIFE, DEATH, AND PLANNING

Death is a subject that most people find difficult to talk about, particularly their own. As a member of the Maryland legislature, I've found people more willing to discuss tax hikes, gang wars, or raw sewage spills than this universal biological fact. Even bringing up the subject often brands the speaker as morbid.

Our fascination with violence in books, television, and movies is well documented. Some have suggested that we like to experience death at a safe distance, as in a murder mystery or slasher flick. We're open to it as long as we can control it—by closing the book or turning off the picture.

Our euphemisms for death are numerous: the grim reaper, deep six, big sleep, dirt nap, buying the farm, kicking the bucket, pushing up daisies, worm food. Talking about it in euphemisms and slang diverts our attention from the cold hard facts.

But when death gets personal, it isn't so easy. It's certainly true that we're delaying death by living longer. When I started in medicine, it was unusual to see patients in their nineties. Yet during a recent emergency room shift, I counted six patients older than 90, and two over 100 years of age. It used to be that the ER staff would buzz when a patient older than 90 would appear. That was a big deal. Now it's routine.

Life can be sustained and the quality of life too. It is said that "60 is the new 40," and nowadays people often get to have two or three careers. Folks don't wind down at age 65; many are just getting started on something new. But death is still waiting for us all at the end of the road.

By the time we reach middle age, most of us have experienced the painful loss caused by the death of a friend or family member. Yet few of us have witnessed someone dying or even seen a dead body that wasn't embalmed and cosmetically presented. In this respect we differ dramatically from prior generations.

There can be advantages to opening our eyes to death.

I get to do frequent talks on this subject, and at these, I always ask audience members to hold up their hand if they have ever been present when someone took their last breath (not counting professional medical experiences). It's never been more than 25% of the audience, and often it's just one or two people. I think our modern estrangement from the reality of death and dying accounts for some of our culture's insatiable hunger for details about other people's deaths, particularly if they are violent: beheadings on videotape, mutilating car accidents, serial killers' crimes.

There can be advantages to opening our eyes to death. On a mundane level, there are financial benefits for our families in estate planning and life insurance policies.

On a spiritual level, many religious sages down the centuries have taught that contemplating their own death unlocked the path to spiritual awakening. From ancient times the end of life has inspired sublime poetry and art.

In our own era, when death can be delayed for decades through medical science, there is a further crucial benefit. By looking at the realities of death and dying, we can make choices that will allow us and our loved ones to find the "best of both worlds," where life is prolonged and the inevitable end is as comfortable, conscious, and supported as possible.

Today we are living longer and better. This is due both to major progress in public health and sanitation and to significant medical advances in diagnostic tests, treatments, devices, pharmaceuticals, and biotechnology. Sometimes we forget how far we've come in such a short time.

For example, years ago when I was a medical resident, getting a CAT scan almost required an act of Congress (and PET scans and MRIs had yet to be developed). There weren't many machines available, maybe only a few for an entire city. Plus, the scans that came back were primitive. I recall seeing brain scans consisting of about six pixels, each the size of one's thumbnail. Nonetheless, we physicians were fascinated with the cutting-edge technology. Today, meticulously detailed CAT scans are routine and done everywhere, including doctors' offices.

Consider the advances in the care of newborns. In 1963 President John F. Kennedy and his wife, Jacqueline, had a son, Patrick Bouvier Kennedy. He was born prematurely, weighing only 4 lbs., 10 oz. Despite the best medical care available, he died 2 days later of respiratory distress syndrome. Today, neonates who weigh less than half that amount regularly survive and thrive.

It used to be fairly rare for someone to survive a heart attack. Only 30 to 40 years ago, treatment consisted primarily of oxygen, pain medicine, and bed rest. Today's world offers clot-busting drugs, medicines to stop fatal arrhythmias, implantable pace-makers, and cardiac surgery. Heart attacks, once a harbinger of imminent death, are now treated aggressively, and many patients live on for decades.

Certain cancers, once fatal, are now routinely treated. For example, lymphoma survivors are common as a result of the evolving field of immunotherapy. Childhood leukemias, both acute lymphocytic leukemia and acute myelogenous leukemia, now have survival rates from 50% to 80%. A few years ago, children with those diseases died quickly and painfully.

But all this progress also created a limbo state. Our bodies can be made to live longer, but when does brain death occur? It's easier to support the plumbing (heart, lungs, kidneys, blood vessels) than to keep the brain functioning at peak level.

Yet even in brain function, progress is being made. Recent advances in hypothermia (lowering body temperature) suggest that there are ways to protect the brain when circulation fails. A brain deprived of blood or oxygen for 4 to 6 minutes undergoes irreparable damage. But with a lower body temperature the brain can enter a state of hibernation, and recovery is possible when the temperature is raised to normal levels. Much more research is needed to define the best ways to induce hypothermia, but again, it's safe to predict that new therapies will emerge.

In the end we will all die of something. And it is not always death that we fear but rather the unknown process of dying. How will I meet my end? Will I be in pain? Will death come swift and sure? Or will it drag out, slow and miserable? We can't know in advance.

HOW CAN WE KNOW THE RIGHT CHOICE?

*In any moment of decision, the best thing you can
do is the right thing, the next best thing is the wrong
thing, and the worst thing you can do is nothing.*
—THEODORE ROOSEVELT

In January 2006 Ariel Sharon, the prime minister of Israel, suffered a massive stroke. He was rushed to the hospital, where he underwent three brain surgeries over the following days. His life was saved, but despite the best available care in the world, he never regained consciousness. Eventually he had major bowel and heart operations as well as treatments for kidney infection and pneumonia. The therapies succeeded, the years rolled by, and Sharon still did not regain consciousness.

Was there ever a chance that Mr. Sharon would return to a semblance of normal life? Was he getting "care," or had he become simply a collection of organs that were kept going by artificial means? Round-the-clock nursing managed each of his bodily functions including tube feeding and waste collection. He was turned regularly to prevent bedsores from developing. When his kidneys failed, he was put on dialysis. Finally, after 8 years in a comatose state, he died.

There is no way to know how much this cost, but in the United States such care would run at least $250,000 per year. So the total for 8 years would exceed $2 million. Apart from the human issues, we have to ask if this is the best way to spend those health care dollars.

Sharon's case is a dramatic and well-known one. We may think that he got this care only because he was a prominent and well-connected person, and there is some truth to that. But similar dramas are taking place every day throughout the United States in every hospital and every nursing home. Modern medicine has put some people into a health care limbo where, like Ariel Sharon, they hover between life and death. This condition can persist for years. A visit to any nursing home will provide numerous examples.

Who knows what these patients are thinking or feeling? How can we know what hurts and what is helpful? Is there a way to know how they would like to be taken care of? How can we best prepare for unpredictable situations?

Diagnosing "brain death," as in Sharon's case, has now become standardized. Once a diagnosis of brain death has been properly declared, there is no reasonable possibility of a patient recovering function.

However, even the best doctors cannot predict with certainty the outcome in any given medical case, especially when dealing with advanced complex illness. Individuals respond differently to treatment. Infections and cancerous growths are often unpredictable. New therapies are continually being discovered. A condition that's currently untreatable may become treatable in a few years.

To begin our exploration of what the dying process may entail and how advanced planning can help in difficult situations, I'm going to share some stories. The names and other identifiers have been changed. All are based on my real-life experience as a physician. They are not always easy to read, but they are accurate descriptions of what happens in today's medical world. Each illustrates a different aspect of end-of-life care and the decisions surrounding it, and each is followed by a discussion of the relevant aspects of advance directives.

TWO PERSONAL EXPERIENCES THAT CHANGED MY LIFE

I always liked those moments of epiphany—
when you have the next destination.
—BRAD PITT

I remember the first time I saw a dead person. It was in 1970 at Highland General Hospital in Oakland, California. A friend of mine was on the straight-and-narrow path to go to medical school and become a doctor, something he'd always planned to do. In order to increase his chances of acceptance to med school, he decided to volunteer at a local hospital emergency room.

I, on the other hand, was ending my college career at the University of California at Berkeley without a clear direction. I was a history major but had done well in high school science classes. I was open to new experiences, so when Robert mentioned his plan and invited me to join him, I accepted.

Our duties consisted of bringing coffee to patients and staff, running blood tubes to the lab, and generally doing little tasks to help the place run better. For me, it was the first time I ever had the chance to chat with a doctor without being a patient. One doctor took a few minutes to explain the concept of an EKG, and I was fascinated and inspired by seeing the graphic traces of electrical activity from the human heart. In that moment, I first thought of becoming a doctor. Medicine looked like the combination of scientific skills and humanitarian values that was right for me.

One evening an ambulance screeched to a halt at the ER entry, and the crew wheeled in a middle-aged woman undergoing cardiopulmonary resuscitation (CPR). The ER became a flurry of activity. I stood in the back and peered between the nurses, doctors, and other staff as they tried to revive the patient. After about 30 minutes, it was clear that the resuscitation effort had failed. The lead doctor halted the proceedings and noted the time of death.

Just as quickly as it had filled with people and machines, the room now emptied. During the few minutes before a nurse aide came to clean the body and transport it to the hospital morgue, I found myself alone with the deceased. I stood in the corner for a minute and then slowly approached the gurney that held the body. I looked at the woman and tried to discern the difference between life and death. After some hesitation, I reached out and gently touched her. No response. Again, and no response. I don't know why I did this. For some reason, her obvious condition was not obvious to me. She looked fine, and yet she was dead. Before I left the treatment room, I silently thanked her for allowing me to be present at her passing.

> You ever wonder what a Martian might think if he happened to land near an emergency room? He'd see an ambulance whizzing in and everybody running out to meet it, tearing the doors open, grabbing up the stretcher, scurrying along with it. "Why," he'd say, "what a helpful planet, what kind and helpful creatures." He'd never guess we're not always that way; that we had to, oh, put aside our natural selves to do it. "What a helpful race of beings," a Martian would say. Don't you think so?
> —ANNE TYLER, THE ACCIDENTAL TOURIST

A second experience concerned my stepfather, Max Mont. He was a remarkable individual. He married my mother when I was 9 years old. Max devoted his life to social change. He read widely and was fully informed on world history, politics, and culture. As a leader in the labor union movement in Los Angeles, he worked for the rights of exploited farmworkers and garment workers and for fair housing and employment laws in California. He built coalitions between disparate groups, and he was an integral part of many steps toward social progress from the 1950s to the 1980s.

As an adolescent Max had been stricken with rheumatic fever that damaged his heart valves. Over the years the damage increased, and Max underwent several major cardiac operations, including a mitral valve replacement. He took excellent care of himself, watching his diet and weight, never smoking or drinking.

But eventually the effect of the surgeries, medications, and recurrent illnesses took their toll. A massive hemorrhage required that one kidney be removed. Within months the other kidney failed, and Max went on dialysis.

Dialysis limited Max as it does all patients. Going to a center three times a week for several hours at a time was exhausting and boring. Max noticed that his mind was starting to fail as well as his body. His memory and alertness faded. He was sleeping more and found that concentrating on a task had become impossible. He could no longer stay focused enough to read or write. For a man who had lived such an active life of the mind, this was devastating.

By that time, I had left California and moved to Maryland. I had been a doctor for more than 15 years. My wife, Shelley, and I had started our family, and I was busy at work as chairman of the Emergency Medicine Department at a large suburban hospital.

One day Max called to tell me that he had made the decision not to return to dialysis. He knew that stopping dialysis would mean the end, and he wanted me to come to Los Angeles to be with him.

When I arrived, my mother and Max and I had a long talk. He looked gaunt and exhausted. He explained that for him life was no longer worth living. He couldn't do anything except stay in bed, sleeping through most of each day. It would take all his strength to rouse himself from his stupor for a few minutes, and then he'd collapse again. Dialysis had worn him out, and he could see that the course of his life would be relentlessly downhill. He knew there was no recovery possible, just more of the same, gradually becoming worse. He wanted to make some decisions while he was still capable.

The next week was intense. Max's family and closest friends came to the bedside to pay their respects. Sometimes, they just sat by, and sometimes they discussed old times. There were both tears and laughter. My mother and I managed the flow of people. By the fifth day, the flow of visitors diminished to a trickle, and toward the end, just the two of us took care of Max.

As the toxins in his blood built up, his waking moments decreased dramatically. Max was more often somnolent than alert. He stopped eating, only occasionally requesting sips of water. We had some codeine pain pills and Valium, and we gave these to Max when he was in pain or became agitated. He began to slide in and out of awareness, but we always kept him as comfortable as possible. We stayed with him continuously, and his last days and hours were peaceful. At the end, his breathing became slower and shallower, slower and shallower. We weren't quite sure when he would take his last breath, but finally it was clear that he was dead.

Max had made arrangements to have his body donated to UCLA Medical School. We hoped that a researcher would learn something from his diseased heart and the condition of his artificial valve that could help other patients in the future.

When my mother and I finished saying our final goodbyes, we called UCLA, and a team arrived to take him away.

Max gave me much, not only in life, but in his death as well. I reflected on his process of dying, so different from the intense activity I knew as a physician. In the hospital, we struggled to keep people going, often long past the time that we knew would offer any hope of meaningful recovery. People died tied to machines and monitors, in the company of strangers, with loved ones in the waiting room.

I often was the one who had to go out and break the bad news. Sometimes there were intensely emotional reactions. I understood this when the death was unexpected or sudden, but it struck me as odd that people would become hysterical when the deceased had been suffering from advanced cancer or clearly terminal heart failure.

This was in stark contrast to what I experienced at home with Max. His death was calm, reassuring, and natural. He had time to say his farewells, and he died at home with family. For those left behind, his death gave us a chance to tell him goodbye, to let go of him gradually. It somehow helped to make the pain of his loss more bearable.

Sometimes, as with the woman who died in that Oakland ER, there are no choices available. People tried their best to save her life, and her loved ones had to deal with the suddenness of their loss as best they could. But when the disease or injury allows us a choice, as in Max's case, it is helpful to have considered these issues in advance of the crisis.

MY DOG GOT BETTER CARE THAN MY MOTHER

America's health care system is neither healthy,
caring, nor a system.
—WALTER CRONKITE

Americans say they love their families, but sometimes it seems like they love their pets more. This was brought home to me as a Maryland state legislator, a role in which I served for 24 years.

Proposed legislation about animals invariably brought out an avalanche of passionate constituent interest. One year there was a bill about allowing acupuncturists to treat animals. This was not just for pets but for horses and farm animals as well. It was the horse breeding and racing industry—big in Maryland—that was pushing for this. In some cases, these racehorses were worth a lot of money, and their owners and trainers wanted every possible treatment available for them. Veterinarians had concerns and opposed the bill. Acupuncturists, of course, favored it, and so the issue became a classic turf war about money. Who would get to treat the animal and bill the owner? The deciding factor was citizens who overwhelmingly wanted that care option for their pets. Letters, emails, faxes, and phone calls poured in. We legislators heard more about animal acupuncture that year than almost any other issue. Eventually, a compromise was worked out whereby a vet had to see the animal once before it could be treated by an acupuncturist, and so this conflict ended well. This episode taught me about how much people are willing to get involved when they feel that their autonomy and individual rights to make medical decisions are threatened.

A dog's life stages are something like ours, only compressed into fewer years. There's puppyhood, then adult years of productive activity, and then eventual deterioration. A dog goes through this in 9 to 15 years, but we can see all the phases mirroring our own.

I've given many talks about end-of-life care, and it's always an interesting experience. First, I wonder if anyone will show up. Given the range of diversions available, who'd want to come and hear a talk about death, dying, and end-of-life care? I try to be entertaining, engaging, and even humorous but also informative and sensitive.

I allow plenty of time for audiences to add their comments and stories. I try to emphasize that we all need a safe place to talk about these issues. This is a hard topic but one that almost all of us have reflected on in one way or another. Often someone raises a hand and says, "My dog got better care than my mother." The person then says how it became apparent that the dog was suffering more and enjoying life less, that a variety of debilitating conditions had set in, and that a veterinarian had finally suggested euthanizing the pet, euphemistically known as "putting it to sleep" or "putting it down." It was a difficult and emotional decision, but once made, it was

If you don't choose to define your medical care, it will be done for you, and all sorts of things can happen that may not be to your liking.

clearly the right one. The time had come. The dog was loved and held, and the final act was done with sensitivity and care.

The same person would go on to say that their mother, on the other hand, went through years of suffering, tears, and medical tests and procedures. No one wanted to say when enough was enough, and nobody was sure what to do or when to do it or who would decide.

Clearly, there's a difference between human life and that of an animal. The key difference in this context is that owners make the choice for a pet and humans can make choices for themselves. And if you don't, all sorts of things can happen that may not be to your liking.

THE STORY OF ALBERTA COLE: NOT DECIDING IS A DECISION

It hath often been said, that it is not death,
but dying, which is terrible.
—Henry Fielding

The following story is not one that I've sensationalized for this book. It's normative, routine, something that is occurring every hour of every day throughout the US health care system. What happened to Alberta can happen to you or someone you love. The question to keep in mind is this: Would you want this for yourself?

When I met Alberta Cole, she was a 92-year-old patient in a nursing home. Born in West Virginia, she and her husband moved to Baltimore after the Second World War when he took a job at the Bethlehem Steel mills. She raised three children and was the proud grandmother of six. A homemaker until her last child moved out, she went back to school to become a bookkeeper. When her husband fell seriously ill with emphysema in the 1990s, Alberta began working from home to care for him. Finally, in 2000 he died.

Alberta continued to live in her modest three-bedroom family home in a working-class neighborhood, but she was becoming increasingly infirm. In 2008 Alberta fell in the bathroom. Unable to get up, she lay on the floor for 2 days until her daughter Mary came to check on her and called 911. She arrived in the ER bruised, dehydrated, and with a hip fracture. A CAT scan of the head showed a small stroke.

Alberta's course in the hospital was difficult. She became agitated in the evenings, something the staff recognized as "sundowning." This term refers to elderly patients who, when away from their familiar home environment, become disoriented and confused at night. Eventually Alberta was discharged to a rehabilitation program in the hospital.

Through her hospital course, her children visited. Daughter Mary, herself in her late sixties, lived in Baltimore and came most often. Her son, Paul, and other daughter, Clare, lived out of town and visited when they could.

The hospital staff ascertained that Alberta did not have an advance directive, and they offered her the forms. But she was too distraught by her pain and disorientation to complete them. Her children doubted that it was necessary. After all, hadn't the doctors and nurses done all they could for Alberta? Wouldn't that continue to be the case?

Eventually Alberta was able to go home, and a visiting nurse was arranged for Mondays, Wednesdays, and Fridays. Alberta's mobility was impaired, and she struggled to move around the house or complete basic chores such as shopping. She became increasingly disheveled and withdrawn. On one visit the nurse observed that Alberta looked weak and pale and had a fever. She called for a private ambulance that took Alberta to the ER.

The ER staff noted that Alberta had multiple problems, the main one being a urinary tract infection. In addition, she had early signs of skin breakdown on her lower back, a consequence of too much sitting. And perhaps worst of all, Alberta showed definite signs of increasing dementia. She was now 80 years old. She knew her name and that she lived in Baltimore but could not give her street address. She knew she was in a hospital but didn't know its name, even though she had been there many times before when taking care of her husband. She didn't know the date, day of the week, or year.

This hospitalization lasted 4 days. Alberta received intravenous antibiotics, physical therapy, and a complete mental health evaluation. It was very difficult to assess the state of her competency to make decisions. Finally, she was stable enough for discharge. But to where could she be safely discharged?

Although Alberta insisted on returning home, her daughter Mary felt that was too risky. Lacking the resources to care for Alberta in her own home, Mary tried to persuade her mother to go to an assisted living center, assuming an affordable one could be found. The other siblings were not available to discuss it. Ultimately Alberta's persistence won out, and she was discharged home with careful instructions, home care with an aide, and a visiting nurse, all arranged with some difficulty by the hospital's social work department.

But this lasted only a few weeks. Alberta did not fare well. Her home aide and visiting nurse tried to persuade her to make a doctor's visit, but Alberta was increasingly hostile and resistant. She had angry outbursts, and once she even took a swing at the nurse.

Another visit to the ER ensued when the aide found Alberta collapsed in her bedroom. The paramedics called in to the hospital, using the medical shorthand "LOL FOF," which means "little old lady, found on floor." That abbreviation is a stark indication of the frequency of patients in similar circumstances.

This led to a 10-day hospitalization. A CAT scan showed multi-infarct dementia, meaning many small strokes had taken their toll on the brain. Alberta's heart, lungs, and digestive system were functioning normally, but she again had a urinary tract infection. Intravenous fluids and antibiotics were given, in addition to anti-anxiety medications to manage her frequent outbursts. Sometimes at night restraints were used to keep Alberta from falling out of bed. One is known, pleasantly enough, as a Posey jacket. (Posey is a brand name that has taken on universal use, like Kleenex for tissue or Xerox for copying.) It's actually a vest that ties the patient to the bed. This is a particularly unpleasant precaution, both for patients and staff.

A social work consultant and a psychiatric consultant were requested, but before those consultations could happen, Alberta suffered a cardiac arrest while being taken for an X-ray.

Alberta's code status had never been determined. She was not wearing a bracelet indicating "DNR," which stands for "do not resuscitate," meaning no cardiopulmonary resuscitation. Her chart was not marked in any way that has become standard when end-of-life decisions have been made. Because she was not designated DNR, by default she became a "full code" patient.

Since staff was present, CPR was started. This involved a hard thump to the chest, followed by cardiac compressions. Most people know what cardiac compressions are, at least from having seen them done on TV, where it's quick and tidy and most people recover. That's not how it is in real life. Here's what actually happens.

To start, both hands are placed on the sternum (breastbone), and in a rocking motion, the heel of the hand depresses the sternum. This helps compress the heart and keep the blood circulating. It also leads to broken ribs at the point where the ribs join the breastbone. Sometimes when doing CPR, you can feel the ribs snap and crack and then crunch on each succeeding chest compression.

An oxygen mask was placed on Alberta's face while preparations were made for intubation. This involves putting a round plastic tube about 18 inches long and three-fourths of an inch wide into the patient's windpipe. First, any dentures or false teeth are removed. Then a laryngoscope is used, a metal tool about 6 inches long and 2 inches wide that pulls open the mouth, sweeps the tongue aside, and widens the oral cavity so the operator (usually a physician, sometimes a respiratory therapist) can see the patient's vocal cords. Sometimes patients vomit during the procedure, so suction equipment is used to remove the chunks and liquid. Sometimes medications are given by vein that paralyze the patient. This is done when the patient is awake or when their jaw is clenched tightly or when their anatomy makes the procedure difficult. Sometimes intubation happens quickly and easily. At other times, it's a trying and difficult process. Once the vocal cords are visible, the operator swiftly jams the tube between them into the windpipe, and the tube's outside end is connected to a ventilator.

The tube in Alberta's windpipe safeguarded her airway and delivered oxygen, but the tube also made it impossible for her to speak. On top of her baseline dementia, the medications administered to ease pain and anxiety, as well as the side effects of other drugs, clouded her mind even further. There was no way to communicate with Alberta or to find out what she was thinking or feeling.

She was transferred to the intensive care unit (ICU). She spent 3 days there and made a slow recovery. The following is a description of basic procedures that are standard practice in ERs and ICUs.

A catheter tube was inserted into the bladder, both to monitor urine output and to prevent self-soiling. This involves threading a lubricated plastic tube about the diameter of a soda straw up through the urinary tract into the bladder. This is a relatively easy procedure, especially in a female patient. It can be more difficult with male patients if the catheter has to pass through an enlarged prostate gland. For any patient, it is an invasive and uncomfortable experience.

Nutrition was given to Alberta through a plastic tube that was inserted through her nose and down into her stomach. I've placed plenty of these, and while not a particularly difficult procedure, patients hate it. We use nasal spray first to shrink the tissues inside the nose, and anesthetic lubricants can ease the passage; but no matter how it's done, it's a tough procedure to endure. Infrequently the nasogastric (NG) tube goes into the windpipe or coils up in the patient's esophagus. Because of this, after every procedure, steps are taken to ensure that the tube is correctly positioned. If incorrectly placed, the procedure must be repeated until done successfully.

Intravenous medications and fluids of all types were given to Alberta and carefully balanced to help recovery and avoid complications. To give fluids intravenously, an IV is established by pushing a needle into a patient's vein, sliding the tube (cannula) over the needle into the vein, taping the tube down, and then removing the needle. Many of us have been on the receiving end of IVs when giving blood or getting fluids or medicine by vein, so we know what it's like to be jabbed by a needle. Like all procedures, sometimes this goes quickly and easily, sometimes not. With elderly patients who have been in the hospital before, it often becomes increasingly difficult to find a good vein. Nurses are adept at locating veins; and while the arms or hands are first choices, sometimes IVs are placed in the feet or legs, or the superficial veins of the neck. Thankfully new techniques are becoming available. For example, trained staff can use portable ultrasound machines to find veins that would otherwise be impossible to locate. But when no sites are found, then more invasive procedures are needed. More on that below.

On day 4 in the ICU, the tube in the windpipe was removed, and Alberta went to the step-down unit.

Alberta was debilitated: her heart, kidneys, and liver had been damaged. These organs were functioning but in a limited way. Her level of awareness was impossible to gauge, but it was becoming obvious that the right side of her body was weaker than the left. The neurologist's note pointed out that this meant the left side of her brain (which controls the right side of the body) had been damaged by a stroke. This also meant that Alberta's use of language was limited, as the location of that function is also in the left side of the brain. Hence, communication, already difficult, became almost impossible.

Liquid nutrition was ordered. At first, this was given via the NG tube, but a tube like that cannot be left in longer than a few days. Now the decision was made to place a G-tube. The "G" stands for "gastric," meaning stomach. Alberta was taken to the operating room. There the surgeon cut a hole in the abdominal wall directly into the stomach. The feeding tube was pushed in and held in place by an internal balloon. Once secured, liquid nutrition can be poured directly into the stomach via the G-tube, allowing the NG tube to be removed.

By day 8 it was time to decide where to send Alberta next. The utilization review (UR) process was beginning. UR brings in insurance companies and their in-hospital representatives (usually nurses) to review the care of patients. Their goal is to shorten hospital stays, limit procedures, and thus reduce their financial exposure. If a patient stays in the hospital too long, the insurance company may refuse to pay for the extra days, meaning that the hospital has to absorb the costs. Sometimes this amounts to thousands of dollars. The hospital counters this process with its own UR committee. This committee does battle with the insurance companies if it disagrees with the company's payment denial. In the best of circumstances, the UR nurse and UR committee cooperate with the patient's attending physician, the person most responsible for the patient's care. The attending physician is, in turn, pushed by several competing forces: the patient's and the family's needs and resources, fear of liability for any wrong decision, and self-interest in getting paid. This tug-of-war is a daily activity in US hospitals.

The hospital's social work team got involved, as it invariably does in this sort of case. Alberta's family was contacted. Mary, the oldest, felt her mother just wanted to "die in peace." But Paul wasn't sure. Clare, who up to this point had left most decisions to

Mary, suddenly became concerned. She insisted that her mother "get the best of care; everything should be done to save her." Clare forcefully pushed her case and implied that she would consider hiring an attorney to make sure this was done. Because of her intense efforts, Alberta's status continued as full code.

In the meantime, several local nursing homes were contacted, and on day 10 of this hospitalization, a bed was found for Alberta. A private ambulance company transported her there from the hospital.

To pay for the nursing home, both Medicare (the federal program for seniors) and Medicaid (the federal program for people with low income) were contacted. Alberta's assets were too great for her to qualify for Medicaid. Thus, the "spend down" process began. Alberta's assets, accumulated over a lifetime, were slowly depleted so that she would eventually be poor enough to qualify for Medicaid. What might have been an inheritance evaporated quickly, as care in a nursing home costs thousands per month.

In the nursing home, Alberta received as good of care as was possible, meaning that it was inconsistent. The nursing home was also under continuous financial pressures. It struggled to attract and retain quality staff. When staff members were good, they were very good; but when they were bad, they could be incompetent or uncaring.

Alberta's days consisted of lying in bed. She had to be turned frequently to avoid bedsores. A word about bedsores. Bedsores develop when the skin breaks down into red areas where pressure has restricted blood flow. Bedsores can become actual open wounds. They can vary from the size of a dime to several inches across. Bedsores can become infected, draining pus, and these infections can take weeks to months to cure, if they can be cured at all. When all else fails, skin grafts may be required to close the open wound, but this doesn't always work.

Bedsores are something every nursing home and chronic care facility struggles to avoid in its patients, but sometimes these are unavoidable. Even Christopher Reeve, the superstar actor who suffered total paralysis from the neck down and who had the very best care money could buy, eventually developed bedsores that contributed to his death.

The nursing staff did all they could to keep Alberta from developing bedsores, but they appeared anyway. Medications and bandages were applied, and although the sores did not get bigger, they didn't shrink either.

On good days, Alberta was taken by wheelchair and placed in the hallway. She would sit and stare at the traffic of patients, family, and staff. Often she'd fall asleep in the chair, slump over, and then be taken back to her room. Or she'd be placed in the TV room, lined up with other patients in front of the TV tuned to daytime game shows or soap operas.

Even Christopher Reeve eventually developed bedsores.

She wore a diaper and needed to be cleaned two to four times per day. Family visits from Mary were daily at first, until this became too demanding for her because of her own medical problems. Paul tried to come weekly, and usually did on Saturdays, spending an hour with his mother. Clare came intermittently, sometimes not for a month or two, and then, if in town, daily for a few days. During these visits, she'd want to meet with the nursing director and Alberta's doctor to go over details of her mother's care plan.

Over the next 6 months, Alberta became increasingly immobile. Her joints became stiff, especially her right arm and leg. These limbs developed contractures, meaning that they slowly became frozen in place, in a flexed position. Alberta was bedridden 24 hours a day.

A urinary catheter had now been in place for weeks. As so often happens, a urinary tract infection developed. This was first evident when Alberta's body temperature spiked with a low-grade fever and the staff noticed that the urine in the collection bag looked cloudy. Alberta's doctor prescribed antibiotics, and these were added to her medication regimen. But her condition did not improve, and one evening Alberta's blood pressure dropped.

Paramedics were called to the nursing home, and the ambulance arrived at 11 p.m. After several jabs, an IV line was placed, fluids given, and Alberta was taken to the ER.

In the ER the nursing staff performed numerous blood and urine tests. After the doctor's examination, X-rays and an EKG were ordered, and fluids and antibiotics were given by vein. However, Alberta's veins were fragile and bruised, and the veins "blew," meaning that fluid was going into the soft tissues around the IV site and not into the bloodstream. Therefore, the ER doctor decided to place a central line, a large IV inserted directly into a large vein located deep below the skin. This would ensure that fluids and medicines were going to the right place.

The three most common areas to insert a central line are the groin (femoral vein), neck (jugular vein), and chest (subclavian vein). In Alberta's case, the doctor chose the subclavian route. The skin on her right upper chest was prepped with an antiseptic solution and then numbed with an injection of lidocaine. Using sterile technique and with careful attention to avoid puncturing vital organs, the doctor first probed the chest with a large needle until the correct vein was punctured. The doctor detects this when blood quickly fills the syringe. Then the syringe is removed, and a metal guide wire is inserted through the needle. The needle is then withdrawn over the guide wire. The skin is then nicked open with a scalpel at the point where the wire enters the skin. A stiff plastic tube (called a dilator) is passed over the guide wire to spread open the tissues to create a wider hole in the vein. The dilator is removed, usually with a gush of blood, leaving a tubular track in its place. This allows the intravenous catheter to be advanced over the guide wire into the vein. The catheter is then stitched into place. This procedure is commonly done in ERs, and I have done this hundreds of times. Sometimes it goes quickly and easily, and the whole procedure takes less than 20 minutes. Sometimes it is difficult and requires repeated searching for the vein. And sometimes there are complications, such as puncturing an artery or a lung. Sometimes a day or two later the patient develops an infection.

With Alberta's central line in place, fluids and medicines were given, and blood was drawn for more testing. After three hours, all the test results were back. These confirmed the diagnosis of a urinary tract infection that had spread to the bloodstream. An hour later the ER physician and Alberta's regular doctor discussed the case and decided to admit Alberta to the hospital. Because the hospital was nearly full, Alberta stayed in the ER for 10 more hours until her bed was ready. She was not aware of the delay; in fact, she did not seem to be aware of anything going on around her.

Because her infection was caused by bacteria that had become resistant to routine antibiotics, more advanced antibiotics were needed. Drug resistance is a real problem for many reasons, including overuse of antibiotics and also recurrent infections in patients who are in and out of hospitals and nursing homes. Nonetheless, during the next 3 days, Alberta's condition gradually improved. On day 4 of this hospitalization, Alberta was without fever and back to baseline function, meaning lying in bed, moaning occasionally, asleep most of the time, and sometimes restrained to prevent her from pulling out tubes.

Back when I was a resident physician in training in the 1970s, I often worked in the ICU. I remember an elderly man, severely ill and chronically debilitated. He was dying of heart, lung, and kidney failure with all their complications. He was on a ventilator. He was very weak, but every day, mustering all his strength and will, he would slowly move his right hand from his side up to his neck, where the plastic airway tube was connected to his tracheotomy (a hole in the front of his neck into the trachea where the tube was inserted). This would take hours, as his hand moved inch by inch. When he'd reach the tube, he'd work to disconnect it.

He wanted to end his suffering, and this suicide attempt was the only way he could communicate his wish. After the first few times of his agonizing effort, the staff realized what was happening. As soon as his hand neared the tube, a nurse or resident physician would run over, pull his hand down to foil his attempt, and the process would start all over again. This patient's attending physician was famous for never "giving up" on his patients. He subjected them to every conceivable treatment, long past any hope of recovery. It was as if he considered stopping treatment—no matter how painful or invasive—to be a professional defeat. Of course, after a couple of weeks of this tragic performance, nature took its course, and the man died.

Because there was no direction in Alberta's case, she was kept alive through two more episodes like the one above. One involved another urinary tract infection, and the other resulted from her bedsores (now large and draining yellow foul-smelling pus). Each required a hospital admission, a central line, and intravenous drugs. There was one brief cardiac arrest, from which she was resuscitated with electrical cardioversion. Eventually she developed pneumonia and again was sent to the hospital. After a day in the ICU, her heart stopped beating. Because her code status was not clear or specified, full CPR was given. Multiple electric shocks, medications, and chest compressions with broken ribs failed to revive her. After 20 minutes, the code was "called" (meaning ended), and Alberta was declared dead.

Twenty-two months had elapsed from her first hospitalization to the last one. From an economic perspective, the hospital costs exceeded $190,000, and nursing home care ran about $6,000 per month. The total, well over $400,000, was much more than Alberta had spent on health care expenses during all the previous years of her life.

More importantly, what was the human cost? Is there a way to quantify Alberta's suffering? She underwent multiple invasive procedures and their complications. She endured numerous transfers between home, ER, operating room, ICU, step-down unit, and nursing home. Through it all she was unable to understand what was happening and unable to communicate her thoughts and feelings. Is that what we would want for ourselves and our loved ones? What are the alternatives?

Alberta's story is typical and quite common. As technology advances and as the senior population grows, millions of Americans will be facing similar circumstances.

I found myself doing things to patients that were closer to torture than healing, and I didn't feel good about it.

It breaks my heart to share this story, but there are many Alberta Coles out there, and I've taken care of more than I can count. Sadly, her story could have been even more graphic and painful than I've written it.

When I see a nursing home patient in the ER who has long-standing mental and physical deterioration, I have a spectrum of reactions. First, I want to be helpful and give the patient the best care possible. But what does that mean?

I have to own up to my part in all this. In the past, when I gave talks, I said things like, "We did this procedure" or "A central line was placed." But these actions didn't happen by themselves. Someone orders them, and that someone was me. I was the one who ordered the start of CPR; I was the one who placed the breathing tube; I was the person who did the central line procedure. As a result, I found myself doing things to patients that were closer to torture than healing, and I didn't feel good about it. I feel guilty for doing some of these things. It was that uncomfortable feeling that got me thinking about how better to approach all this.

Sometimes I rationalized: this is the system; I'm part of it; I do my job as best I can. At other times I got angry because of the agony we put patients through, as well as the time, energy, money, and medical talent spent on treatment that neither cures nor comforts. What will I do tomorrow if another Alberta presents for care? The best answer is for each of us to be sure that we don't end up in

Alberta's situation unless that's what we want. But I'm willing to bet that most of us don't.

There was no way to know for sure what Alberta would have wanted. But let's change the story. Let's say that when she was still able and competent, Alberta had completed an advance directive shortly after her husband died.

Let's introduce an advance directive into Alberta's story and speculate what might have gone differently for her.

At the beginning, after the first fall, she needed all that the health care system had to offer. Her broken hip had to be repaired. But after that, an advance directive could have prompted her caregivers to ask whether providing additional services would help her or not. Alberta could have specified that she wanted the best of medical care but would allow nature to take its course if she became demented and unable to live a normal life. To start, that would have included no CPR. It could also have included no major invasive procedures such as a central line or a feeding tube. It could have included antibiotics only for routine infections with a good chance of cure. At that point, her advance directive could have stipulated that she wanted routine care with attention paid especially to her comfort.

A key problem for Alberta was that it wasn't clear who was making the medical decisions for her. Given her family dynamics, it would have been logical for Mary, the eldest and closest to her, to be in charge. Mary knew her mother wanted to "die in peace," and this would have lessened the burden and involvement for her siblings. Equally important, Mary could have directed the health care team with what her mother would have wanted or not wanted.

The net result is that Alberta would have died a bit sooner but with far less suffering and consistent with her wishes.

2

Taking Charge

ADVANCE DIRECTIVES AND CHOOSING THE CARE YOU WANT

———

Tennis taught me so many lessons in life. One of the
things it taught me is that every ball that comes to me,
I have to make a decision. I have to accept responsibility
for the consequences every time I hit a ball.
—BILLIE JEAN KING

Each of us will have our own way of facing the end of life. I've dealt with many individuals and families, and no two are alike. The next two chapters tell of two men who chose different approaches, neither of which I would have wanted for myself. But they show the range of feelings and thoughts people have as they approach critical illness.

THE STORY OF MICHAEL MARTINEZ
AND HIS DECISION

Michael Martinez was a personal friend and medical colleague. He was a methodical and passionate man, with four primary interests in life. One was his profession. He had always known he wanted to be a doctor. After graduating from the University of Virginia Medical School, he served in the navy for two years and then completed his training in internal medicine at Johns Hopkins University. Michael was a "doctor's doctor" who set aside time each day for his continuing education, when he studied medical journals and textbooks to make sure he was aware of all the latest scientific findings. He was also a "patient's doctor." His devotion to his patients' care was what we'd all like to see from our physicians. In fact, I learned a lot of both the science and art of medicine from him, and I enjoyed our medical conversations.

His second passion was his 25-foot powerboat. He took meticulous care of his craft, working on it every available weekend. He kept careful maintenance records, as well as a log of every guest and outing. Michael knew the Chesapeake Bay and all its inlets and rivers. He'd cruised from Maryland down the Inland Passage to Florida. He attended boat shows to keep up on the latest gear, and he wrote articles for boating magazines.

His third passion was staying fit. A varsity baseball player in college, he'd always worked out and stayed in shape. He never smoked, drank alcohol, or used any drugs. He was as straight-arrow as they come.

Last, and most important, Michael loved his family. His wife, Carla, was his closest friend and companion. His daughter, Rachel, inherited his interest in science. She worked for a research company and was the mother of two young children.

Michael's symptoms began gradually and with great subtlety. At the start, he noticed that he seemed tired after what had previously been routine exertion. This didn't make any sense to him. He intensified his workout regimen, but the weakness and fatigue only got worse. He developed heartburn after eating, unusual in someone who had always been a robust eater and had no risk factors for acid reflux. Medical work-up was not revealing; routine tests were normal. Michael had access to the best medical specialists, who proposed various theories. He eventually became convinced that his symptoms were the side effects of cholesterol-lowering drugs. He stopped taking the drugs, but the symptoms persisted.

Over the next few months, the symptoms became more pronounced. At least one night a week he would be awakened from a sound sleep by choking spasms and have difficulty catching his breath. On two occasions he had to go to the emergency room before he could resume normal breathing. Michael had an intuition of what was causing his problems, but his suspicion was too horrifying even to share with Carla. More work-ups followed. Again, all routine tests, including CAT scans, were negative, but careful nerve and muscle tests showed deterioration. The diagnostic choices were limited, and as all other diseases were ruled out, only one possibility remained. It was what Michael had feared: amyotrophic lateral sclerosis (ALS).

Commonly known as Lou Gehrig's disease, rare in the population but more common among US military veterans, ALS is a progressive neuromuscular condition that starts in nerve cells in the spinal cord. As these cells die, the muscles they control fail. Eventually most patients are not able to stand or walk, get in or out of bed on their own, or use their hands and arms. In Michael's case, the nerve cells that were the first to go were in his throat, affecting his ability to swallow, chew, and speak. ALS does not affect cognitive function, so patients are completely aware and competent. There is no specific treatment, and average survival after diagnosis is 3 to 5 years. But for reasons no one understands, a small percentage of ALS patients live far longer, surviving for 10, 20, or 30 years after diagnosis.

Michael observed his body's deterioration with scientific attention. He watched the fasciculations (the twitching of muscles in their death throes) that were visible through the skin in his forearms and legs. Michael had taken care of patients with ALS and seen them die. He knew what was in store for him: an inexorable downhill course culminating in death, possibly caused by an inability to breathe.

Almost immediately upon diagnosis, Michael made a decision that he would do nothing to prolong his life. For a while he contemplated suicide but then rejected it as too upsetting for Carla and Rachel. We once even discussed how he would do it. He'd take his boat out into the ocean and throw himself overboard. He joked that he'd caught and eaten lots of fish, so wasn't it about time that he returned the favor?

Instead, Michael slowly and painfully watched his body deteriorate, and he grew more and more despondent. He knew better than most that disease has nothing to do with fairness, but he still resented his fate. He was only 59 years old. He had always taken good care of himself and tried so hard to do good for others.

Michael knew there were options to make his decline more comfortable and to keep him functioning for the longest time possible. Physical therapy could help accommodate his bodily limitations. Speech therapy could help with his increasingly slurred speech. There were assistive devices to help with breathing and communication, and motorized wheelchairs to compensate for the growing deficits in his mobility. His health insurance and veterans' benefits would help cover the costs. Carla, his family, and several friends urged him to make use of these aids, but Michael declined them all. Already his medical practice had become limited to paperwork. Boating was out of the question. Driving and even walking grew progressively more difficult. Finally, he put in for early retirement.

Carla strove to give Michael the best quality of life possible. She still prayed that he would be one of the lucky long-term survivors, but when she considered his situation realistically, she knew he didn't have much time left. Before he became too disabled, they managed a cruise in the Caribbean. Michael was in a wheelchair, and while they couldn't participate in most of the shore excursions, it gave him an opportunity once again to be on the water, to be at one with the sea he loved so much. At home, there were frequent visits from Rachel and the grandchildren, as well as from friends, colleagues, patients, and cousins who came from as far away as Europe to say their farewells.

Michael made a few concessions to prolonging his life. When he could no longer swallow comfortably without choking, he agreed to a gastrostomy tube. Now he took all hydration and nutrition directly into his stomach. When breathing became too difficult, he began using a positive pressure ventilation device called a BiPAP to help move air in and out of his lungs.

His physicians urged him to have a tracheostomy (a hole into the windpipe through the lower neck) so that when the BiPAP no longer provided enough help, he would be able to transition to a full ventilator. They stressed that his mind was as sharp as ever and that although a ventilator would prevent speaking, he could employ computers and other devices to communicate. There were still many avenues open to him for the enjoyment of life. They pointed to the example of Stephen Hawking, the world-renowned physicist who survived more than 30 years with ALS, continuing his distinguished scientific career despite being almost completely paralyzed and on a ventilator.

I remember one discussion I had with Michael. He expressed his deep frustration about the whole situation, a frustration he had never demonstrated but that he shared with me. He had done all the right things, lived a clean life, done good work, and here he was now being pushed around in a wheelchair, needing someone to feed him, wash him, attend to his every bodily need. This too was part of his decision not to drag things out.

I argued that as long as his mind was working, life was worth living. After all, although he was uncomfortable, he wasn't in pain. Of course it would be hard, even humiliating at times, to be a prisoner within a dysfunctional body. But he'd be able to watch his grandchildren grow (and impart his life's wisdom to them), see how the latest election would turn out (would Obama get reelected?), enjoy movies, and play games such as Scrabble. At least, that's what I projected I'd want if I were in his situation. Of course it was much easier opining from the outside than living it from the inside. Who knows what I'd really want if our roles were reversed?

Michael's doctors and his friends respected his decision not to prolong his life, even if they couldn't really understand his reasoning. Why not keep going? But characteristically, Michael had based his decision on what to him was a rational assessment of his situation. If he couldn't do the things he loved—practice medicine, be on his boat, exercise vigorously, and spend quality time with his family—then he didn't want to continue living. To him, these were the most important things in life, and without them, living had no purpose. This perspective was troubling to almost everyone, including Carla. But she and Michael had agreed that they would each honor the wishes of the other in sickness and in health.

Some want the full-court press in end-of-life care. Would you?

As Michael grew weaker, he gave up leaving the house. He spent most days in bed, entertained by science fiction movies on TV. For the last 5 months of his life, Michael needed virtually 24-hour care. This responsibility primarily fell to Carla, until the last 6 weeks when Rachel took family and medical leave from her job so that she could move in with her parents. Friends and family pitched in to support Carla and Rachel with meals, errand running, and companionship.

A turning point came when hospice was consulted. This led to almost daily visits by the staff, something appreciated by both Michael and Carla. Hospice provided a number of important services. First, there were respite times for Carla and Rachel. Second, hospice taught them skills to take care of Michael, making the daily chores of feeding, washing, toilet, etc. easier. Third, hospice provided a medication regimen that relieved some of Michael's worst symptoms. Frequently Michael would experience the agony of "air hunger," the sensation of drowning caused by his inability to draw enough air into his lungs. These episodes were treated by medicines to reduce pain and anxiety, combined with suctioning the airway to clear mucus. The team worked to balance Michael's medications, giving him enough morphine to keep the air hunger at bay, while not sedating him any more than was necessary.

Soon after his diagnosis, Michael had rewritten his advance directive to reflect his current thinking. He stated what he wanted, and then he put Carla in charge. As Michael withdrew, it became Carla's responsibility to handle all the medical decisions. This was difficult and stressful. They'd been married more than 30 years, and she knew her husband better than anyone. She didn't want to lose him a minute sooner than necessary, but as tough as it was, she was determined to do what he had asked of her.

In the final days, Michael was awake for only brief periods. His pulse became rapid, his skin clammy, and his extremities cold. Breathing was labored, and as the oxygen level in his blood fell, his mental function began to deteriorate. Finally, the oxygen dropped so low that his heart was unable to keep working; and with a last gasp and shudder, he died in Carla's arms, 15 months after his diagnosis.

The key for Michael was that he had discussed his concerns and wishes with family and friends, had thought through his decision, documented it in his advance directive, and made sure his wife understood and would do what he wanted. He accomplished this with the first part of an advance directive.

ADVANCE DIRECTIVES: TREATMENT PREFERENCES

"If I know Mom," she said, "she'd have refused any surgery anyhow." "It's true," Amanda said. "Her advance directive basically asked us to put her out on an ice floe if she developed so much as a hangnail."
—ANNE TYLER, A SPOOL OF BLUE THREAD

The first section of the advance directive usually covers what kind of care you want, and it goes by different names. It might be titled "Treatment Preferences," "Living Will," or "Instructions for Health Care." But all these terms refer to the same consideration: What are the basic values and standards you'd like to see applied should you become unable to make decisions for yourself? (figure 2.1).

The Treatment Preferences section gives guidance to physicians and families as they make determinations about the kind of care a person wants. The purpose is to allow people to outline the care that they feel is appropriate for them. The limitation is that it's difficult to anticipate every complexity of specific medical decisions that may arise. For example, one's Treatment Preferences may say, "Keep me comfortable and pain free." But sometimes it can be hard to translate what is "comfortable" and "pain free" into appropriate dosages of sedative or opioid medications. That's why Treatment Preferences work best when the person has also designated a health care agent who holds their medical power of attorney (more about this in chapter 5).

Some advance directive forms include a statement of values. This is the opportunity to offer, in a few sentences of your own composition, something about your goals and wishes during the last part of life.

For example, one person's statement might say, "To me, the life of the mind is the most important thing. If it appears that my mind is not functioning, if I'm not aware of what's going on, if I can't relate to people who are around me, with no chance of re-

Figure 2.1. Decision tree: facing serious illness

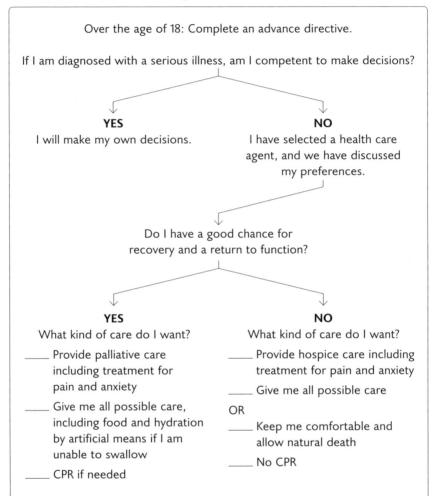

Over the age of 18: Complete an advance directive.

If I am diagnosed with a serious illness, am I competent to make decisions?

YES
I will make my own decisions.

NO
I have selected a health care agent, and we have discussed my preferences.

Do I have a good chance for recovery and a return to function?

YES
What kind of care do I want?

____ Provide palliative care including treatment for pain and anxiety

____ Give me all possible care, including food and hydration by artificial means if I am unable to swallow

____ CPR if needed

NO
What kind of care do I want?

____ Provide hospice care including treatment for pain and anxiety

____ Give me all possible care

OR

____ Keep me comfortable and allow natural death

____ No CPR

covery, then I don't consider prolonging my life to be worthwhile. Just keep me comfortable and pain free, and let nature take its course."

Another person's might read, "I believe in the wholeness of life. Even if I don't appear to be able to comprehend what's going on around me, there still could be consciousness within me. My experience, no matter how it may appear to others, is still my experience, and I value it. Plus, there have been cases where people who seemed to be out of it eventually recovered and continued to enjoy life. You can't tell. So, please keep me alive as long as possible."

In effect, what Michael chose was this: "I've lived a good life, but I don't want to continue to live disabled and unable to enjoy the things that mean the most to me. I know what dying with ALS looks like: it's a long, miserable, drawn-out process, and I don't want that. I'll accept some treatments, but in the end, I don't want to be propped up, paralyzed from the neck down, signaling only with my eyes, with all my bodily functions handled by others. When that time comes, let nature take its course, and I'll die in peace. You may not understand or agree with what I want, but it's my life, and it's what I want that counts."

Following the statement of values, the next section covers specific care situations. Typically, the choices to make come in three categories: do little or nothing; do something; do everything.

EXAMPLE OF TREATMENT PREFERENCE CHOICES

Here's an example, taken from Maryland's "Treatment Preferences" section:

Preference in case of terminal condition.

If my doctors certify that my death from a terminal condition is imminent, even if life-sustaining procedures are used:

1. Keep me comfortable and allow natural death to occur. I do not want any medical interventions used to try to extend my life. I do not want to receive nutrition and fluids by tube or other medical means.

OR

2. Keep me comfortable and allow natural death to occur. I do not want medical interventions used to try to extend my life.

If I am unable to take enough nourishment by mouth, however, I want to receive nutrition and fluids by tube or other medical means.

OR

3. Try to extend my life for as long as possible, using all available interventions that in reasonable medical judgment would prevent or delay my death. If I am unable to take enough nourishment by mouth, I want to receive nutrition and fluids by tube or other medical means.

The California form approaches this slightly differently in a section headed "End-of-Life Decisions." Here's what it says:

I direct that my health care providers and others involved in my care provide, withhold, or withdraw treatment in accordance with the choice I have marked below:

Choice Not To Prolong Life:
_____ I do not want my life to be prolonged if (1) I have an incurable and irreversible condition that will result in my death within a relatively short time, (2) I become unconscious and, to a reasonable degree of medical certainty, I will not regain consciousness, or (3) the likely risks of treatment would outweigh the expected benefits.

OR

Choice To Prolong Life:
_____ I want my life prolonged as long as possible within the limits of generally accepted health care standards.

In addition to these examples, there are many other versions, including ones that come from religious organizations and that reflect their specific value set. However, you can always modify or add to a form or even choose to write your own version. You can include as much detail and be as creative and specific as you wish. For example, you can indicate what kinds of food and entertainment you'd prefer; whom you would like to see or not see; whom you'd want to accompany you on medical visits; whether or not you'd want to go to a nursing facility; whom you'd prefer to take care of your personal hygiene if needed; what room in your house you'd like to spend most of your time in; and so on.

_____

The decision belongs to the person whose life is at stake, not to their family.

_____

Some people choose to identify certain activities or abilities that measure quality of life for them personally. The loss of those capacities can serve as an indicator to their health care agents that heroic measures to prolong life are no longer desired. One example of this might be losing the ability to recognize family members and friends.

An advance directive does not have to limit care in any way. It merely defines the type and degree of care that a person wants. How one answers these questions is entirely personal. The choices made should stem from an individual's understanding of life and its meaning. Let's get into a few of the specifics.

CPR: CARDIOPULMONARY RESUSCITATION

One key decision is whether or not you want CPR. Most people know the basics of CPR, from TV, movies, or first aid courses. In its simplest form, the victim gets airway clearing, mouth-to-mouth breathing, and chest compressions. Sometimes an AED (automated external defibrillator) can be used. These are often found in public places, such as airports, large buildings, and arenas. AEDs, using computer programs, shock the patient's heart and hopefully restore a normal heart rhythm.

The most sophisticated forms of CPR are provided in hospitals by medical staff or in the field by full-level paramedics. In these cases, the patient may be intubated (with a plastic tube inserted into the airway) and get medications by vein such as epinephrine, lidocaine, and atropine. In hospitals these CPR events are called "codes," and one might hear the words "code blue, CCU" over a hospital's public address system. A code can last 5 minutes to an hour, depending on the patient's response to treatment and other factors.

There are dramatic occurrences of recovery after CPR, but unfortunately, despite years of research and study, CPR is still rarely effective. Survival rates from CPR, when it's started in a community setting, average around 4% to 6%. These rates are somewhat higher in hospitals. A few years ago an article in the *New England Journal of Medicine* compared CPR success rates on medical television shows with real-world statistics. Perhaps not surprisingly, staff on the shows ER and *Grey's Anatomy* save more than 75% of their patients. I only wish we could match that record.

The biggest factors in CPR success are the previous health of the victim, the time elapsed between the arrest and onset of CPR, the technique used by the person performing CPR, and the underlying cause of the arrest. For example, a drowning victim who's promptly pulled from a cold lake has a better chance of successfully being revived than an elderly and debilitated victim of a blocked coronary artery.

Interestingly, the practice of how to do CPR has evolved. For many years, experts recommended—and everyone was taught—to "follow the ABCs." That meant "airway," "breathing," and "compressions," and this was the order in which to do things. Millions of practitioners at all levels for decades had this sequence drilled into their heads. We were also carefully instructed to interpose the breath (mouth-to-mouth or with a ventilator bag) between the chest compressions, although for a while it was thought they should be given at the same time.

Then a few years ago, it all changed. Now we are supposed to "take a CAB." The new order became "compressions," "airway," and then "breathing." I hope this change has increased the survival rate, but it's probably too early to tell. But one of my takeaways from all this is that medical dogma can change. Today's ideas, no matter how sacrosanct, may be subject to revision as new information becomes available. Therefore, one's thinking as a physician has to stay flexible. Experts may not know as much as they think they do, and what seems like common sense today may not remain so in the future.

CPR has its place, but I didn't like the feeling I had in the ER when I was the one ordering CPR for a patient who was unlikely to benefit. It was more torture than care. But without an advance directive to guide me, there was little or nothing I could do in the acute care setting of the ER.

A number of hospitals are now using the abbreviation "AND," which stands for "allow natural death." That sounds better to me than "DNR" (do not resuscitate) or "no CPR," the most common ways of denoting that the patient is not to get a full code in the event of cardiopulmonary arrest.

NOURISHMENT AND WATER . . . OR NOT

As the dying process sets in, a person's appetite dwindles. In fact, many experts look at appetite loss in a severely ill person as one of the signs that the end is near. Eating and drinking are basic human activities, surpassed only by breathing in immediate necessity. As the body begins to shut down, the demand for nourishment fades. The body quiets, metabolism slows, and the desire to eat and drink recedes. Sometimes patients only want enough water to keep their lips and mouth moist.

It is debated whether withholding nourishment is painful for a person dying of other medical causes and, therefore, whether it is ethical. This is a complex topic with a spectrum of opinions. Often what to do depends on the specifics of each case.

Let's take the case of a person dying of cancer who has had all possible treatments, but the cancer has spread throughout the body. Appetite is gone, and the person has lost weight, becoming skeletal. There is pain, but it is well controlled with pain medicine. The person is getting weaker every day, with only limited periods of being awake and aware. Breathing is labored, and the person is bedbound. In this case, trying to extend life with fluids is useless and in fact may prolong the agony.

Or consider a young person who has suffered a severe traumatic brain injury. The person is comatose; the EEG is a flat line, and the CAT scan shows that brain tissue has deteriorated and been replaced by fluid. There is no hope of improvement or recovery. However, the rest of the patient's bodily functions work normally. The patient breathes, the heart pumps blood, and the digestive tract processes food. The patient requires constant monitoring and hourly care, turning to avoid bedsores, and physical therapy to minimize limb contractures. In this case, nutrition can prolong the patient's life, sometimes for years. Whether this should be done or not is something that is difficult to decide. If the patient has an advance directive and chose one of the options for nourishment, then the caregivers would know what to do. If the patient had designated a health care agent, then that person could decide. But if nothing had been written and no one designated, then choosing the proper course of action is problematic.

Here's a third case. A patient was injured high in the spinal cord and became paralyzed from the neck down. Unable to move anything below the neck, this person requires daily care for all physical needs. But the patient is awake, alert, conscious, oriented, and can communicate. This person falls into the category of having an end-stage condition, defined as a condition that continues in its present course until death and that has resulted in a loss of capacity and complete physical dependency. In this case, since the patient can make their wishes known, the advance directive would not come into effect. The patient's choice of whether to receive nutrition is the same as any other adult's choice to eat or not. It is rare for such patients to refuse sustenance, but the law protects their right to do so without being subjected to forced feedings.

3

A Different Choice

DO EVERYTHING

─────────

*For I am—or I was—one of those people who pride themselves
on their willpower, on their ability to make a decision and carry it
through. This virtue, like most virtues, is ambiguity itself. People
who believe that they are strong-willed and the masters of their
destiny can only continue to believe this by becoming specialists in
self-deception. Their decisions are not really decisions at all—a real
decision makes one humble, one knows that it is at the mercy of
more things than can be named—but elaborate systems of evasion,
of illusion, designed to make themselves and the world appear to be
what they and the world are not.*

—James Baldwin

THE STORY OF JOSEPH KRANZ AND HIS DECISION

In the previous chapter, Michael Martinez chose limited treatments. Joseph Kranz, whose story follows, made a different set of
choices.

When Joseph's wife, Edith, died from a pulmonary embolism,
the last thing she told him was not to mourn her too long. She
said, "Life is a gift. Take all of it you can. Be there for the family."

Joseph and Edith had had a good life together. They'd been married 50 years and had three children, now grown with families of their own. As a first-generation child of German immigrants, Joseph was a self-made American success story. Raised in a Pennsylvania coal town, he worked hard and was always ready to make the most of his opportunities. He earned his degree in civil engineering at Penn State with the help of the GI Bill, graduating just as the national interstate highway system was beginning construction in the 1950s. He ended his career as the senior partner of a prosperous engineering firm in southern California (home of a massive freeway complex), retiring when he turned 70.

He and Edith had enjoyed another few years together before a broken hip led to the embolism (blockage of a blood vessel by a blood clot) that took her life. Joseph was deeply saddened, but he kept his perspective, and he took Edith's advice to heart. He stayed active, and he increased his charitable work, even endowing the Kranz Pavilion at a local art museum and contributing to various health care charities, including his local hospital.

Joseph enjoyed fairly good health. He hadn't smoked in more than 30 years and drank alcohol in moderation. He'd been diagnosed with high blood pressure at age 50, but this condition was controlled by medication. At age 80 he noticed that his legs seemed swollen, and he started having episodes of night sweating. Then he found a small lump in his armpit. It didn't hurt, but it hadn't been there before. He could no longer ignore the symptoms.

Joseph was admitted to the hospital, where he underwent numerous tests and procedures: blood work, imaging scans, bone marrow tests, a biopsy of lymph gland tissue with microscopic analysis, and consultations with various specialists. Finally, his doctor had the diagnosis: lymphoma.

Lymphoma is a cancer of the immune system cells called lymphocytes. There are many types of lymphoma depending on the specific immune cells involved, but it was clear that Joseph's case was advanced.

I got to know Joseph as a close friend of one of his sons who called on me frequently for advice and, at times, for referrals to physician specialists. Most of the time, though, he just wanted to process what was going on with his father and the medical decisions involved. I didn't mind being of service in this way.

Treatment of lymphoma is complicated, and 20 years ago it was much less effective than the newer treatments available today. Joseph was admitted to the hospital and referred to an oncologist. Dr. Patel was guardedly optimistic. She told Joseph that most patients survive more than 5 years, but there was no way to predict what would happen in an individual case. Joseph might do well, but he already was older than most patients with lymphoma.

Prior to beginning chemotherapy, a catheter tube was placed in a large vein in Joseph's chest, creating a special opening (port) located just below the skin. A port can be used to infuse medications without having to find a new vein for each cycle of chemotherapy.

Dr. Patel explained that there would be several cycles of chemo, and that while the medications were balanced to reduce side effects, these were not completely avoidable. As predicted, Joseph's hair fell out, he felt sick and tired, and he had a sore mouth. His family helped him as best they could, and a day nurse was hired to take care of him during the week when everyone was at work.

The experience shook Joseph. For the first time in his life, he was not in control. This brush with his own death frightened him, but it also energized him. He was a fighter; he wasn't going to let the cancer get the better of him. He began to research his medical condition. He pored over the latest studies on lymphoma, its causes and treatments. He found inspiring stories of long-term survivors. He reviewed medical journals, and he began to contact national and international authorities about new therapies. He read about alternative treatments, including vitamin and vaccine therapies. He even investigated cryonics, where a person is kept in a frozen state after death until a cure for their problem can be found, but he decided that this approach was not sufficiently developed . . . yet.

Dr. Patel cautiously suggested that Joseph consider a palliative care program at the hospital and a hospice consultation, both relatively new items at the time.

Since then studies have conclusively demonstrated that terminally ill patients who participate in a palliative care program, even while pursuing aggressive treatment, live longer and have better quality of life than those who wait till the end to get help for their symptoms. But back in the 1990s, this was all new stuff.

Joseph was suspicious. Wasn't "palliative care" just another name for hospice? And wasn't hospice for those who had no chance of recovery? Dr. Patel tried to explain the distinctions, but Joseph wasn't buying it. "It sounds like you're giving up on me," he said. Joseph went through several rounds of therapy over the next two years. When one drug stopped working, Dr. Patel would try another. Joseph was ever hopeful for a new and better treatment, but eventually the lymphoma stopped responding. He continued to pore over news reports and medical journals about his condition. He was willing to try anything.

When Joseph had completed his advance directive, he'd studied the forms carefully. In each case, he chose to prolong his life as long as possible. He didn't want "to pull the plug" because "who knows what treatment might be discovered tomorrow?" He didn't want to miss out on a miracle cure because he'd given up too soon.

Joseph designated his eldest son, Gary, as his health care agent. Gary and his siblings were conflicted. On the one hand, they loved their father deeply, and they treasured the last two years that the chemo had bought them. But on the other hand, they could see the pain and suffering he endured with each round of treatment. Sometimes the cure seemed worse than the disease.

When Gary mentioned his concerns, Joseph was offended. Didn't Gary and the others want him to survive as long as there was a chance for a cure? Were they anxious to get their hands on his money? Gary quickly backed off, assuring his father that he would abide by his wishes to the letter.

Joseph asked about getting a bone marrow transplant, then a cutting-edge therapy with more failure than success, and Dr. Patel was skeptical. A transplant meant finding an acceptable donor, followed by intensive chemo and radiation therapy to wipe out the patient's bone marrow and immune system. Then the new bone marrow would be infused, and it could take weeks or months to gauge the response. During that time the patient would be in isolation, at risk from even the most minor illness or complication. At 84, weakened by years of cancer therapy, Joseph would be unlikely to survive such an intense regimen.

But Joseph was adamant. He called the hospital administrator and reminded him of his donations to the institution. He was willing to go anywhere in the United States where this was done. He wanted this chance, and he was willing to pay for it, even if his insurance wouldn't cover the bill.

Gary and the family were shocked that Joseph was willing to try a difficult experimental treatment that at best might buy him only a few more months of life. Wouldn't it be better for him to die at home or in a hospice than in the hospital undergoing uncomfortable procedures? But they had learned not to question their father's wishes. In his darker moments, Gary wondered if his father's dogged fight for life came from his will to live or from his fear of death.

It was during his last hospitalization that I got a bit more involved. I had gotten to know the family and the whole story. I wasn't making key decisions. Instead, I was an active bystander.

My conversations with Joseph were generally about his life, his attitude toward his condition (anger), and his insistence that "everything be done." He had a tendency to ring the nurse call button incessantly, and he'd let everyone know if the response wasn't quick enough. One of my roles was to calm Joseph down after episodes of his chewing out the staff.

As Joseph was beginning the work-up for the transplant, his condition grew worse. Breathing became more difficult, and a fever set in. Pneumonia, kidney failure, and low blood counts were diagnosed. In critical condition, Joseph was transferred to the ICU. Within a few hours, his blood pressure began to fall as sepsis (widespread bloodstream infection) developed. Infusions to boost his blood pressure, along with broad-spectrum antibiotics, were given.

By the time the rest of the family arrived, Joseph had lapsed into a coma, his breathing maintained by a ventilator. Dr. Patel met with the family, explaining that the sepsis was not responding to treatment; his immune system was too battered. Their father would not regain consciousness or recover sufficiently to undergo the transplant. She advised them to say their goodbyes and remove the ventilator. Gary's younger siblings wanted to follow the doctor's advice. They felt their father had suffered enough. He had fought the good fight, but now it was time to go. Gary hesitated. They gathered at Joseph's bedside in the ICU cubicle, finding space to stand between the machines and monitors. Joseph burned with fever from the advancing infection. His hands and feet were cold and darkening, signs of shock and decreased circulation. But Gary had promised not to "pull the plug." They took turns keeping their ICU vigil until the next afternoon when the sepsis overwhelmed him, and Joseph finally breathed his last.

I watched this process and was distraught. Joseph's last hours were ones of intense suffering. He never really said his goodbyes to his children. The whole effort was an exercise in futility. It was what he wanted, but I promised myself that I wouldn't let that happen to me.

Both Michael and Joseph made decisions I would not have. If I had ALS, was not in pain, and had mental function intact, I believe I'd choose to keep going as long as possible with a tracheotomy, breathing assistance, and every modern device to help me move about and communicate. If I had advanced cancer, I'd take a shot or two at chemo, or even a transplant; but I'd want to know when further treatment was useless, and I'd ask my doctors to be clear about that. Then I'd go home and allow nature to take its course, making sure I was as comfortable as possible for as long as possible. In both these stories, the families would have made different choices for their dying loved one.

Some people want everything, some want to let go, but most of us are in the middle when it comes to wanting medical intervention.

But the decision belongs to the person whose life is at stake, not to the person's family. As a physician, my job is to provide the best information possible without partiality or prejudice. As a legislator, I wanted to ensure that everyone be empowered to make these decisions without undue outside interference. Even if I disagree, I try not to question or to judge but rather to follow the advance directive as closely as possible.

HOW TO DECIDE: WEIGHING PRIORITIES

In a world where every road, after a few miles, forks into two, and each of those into two again, and at each fork, you must make a decision.
—C. S. LEWIS

It is hard to know what to do and when, what procedures might work, and which ones might not be worth the risk. As a clinician, family member, and patient, I find it helpful to divide medical testing and treatments into four categories:

1. High benefit, low risk: this would include laceration repair, fixing of routine fractures, CAT scans to rule out serious disease, as well as preventive measures (diet, exercise, meditation) and standard safety measures (wearing seat belts).

2. Low benefit, low risk: there aren't too many in this category, but it might include taking vitamin supplements or relatively unproven "new age" treatments.

3. High risk, high benefit: here it gets tricky, as it could include bone marrow transplant for leukemia, major cancer surgery, open heart surgery for valve replacement, or organ transplantation.

4. High risk, low benefit: this could include major procedures for purely cosmetic benefit, full CPR in the case of advanced illness, or extended experimental chemotherapy.

Running through all of these considerations are individual factors, such as the age and condition of the patient. A bone marrow transplant for an otherwise healthy young adult with leukemia makes sense, but it would not for a 90-year-old with advanced dementia. Still, when faced with complex medical decisions, we all could benefit from having an approach to help us analyze the pros and cons, the risks and benefits of each.

WHAT ABOUT SURGERY IN OLDER ADULTS?

In the past, surgical procedures on older adults were discouraged and feared. However, new standards have been developed by the American College of Surgeons. These standards have made surgery safer with improved outcomes. Deciding whether a senior should undergo a procedure is one for both the patient and the surgeon to review carefully with these guidelines in mind. If you are an older adult contemplating surgery, you should be sure your surgeon and surgical team are aware of these. A free download from www.facs.org/geriatrics explains it well.

One of the leaders and pioneers in improving the evaluation of surgical treatment for seniors is Dr. Mark R. Katlic. He is the chair of the Department of Surgery and director of the Center for Geriatric Surgery of the Lifebridge Health System in Baltimore, Maryland.

In writing on this subject, Katlic points out that

the continued aging of the population will be perhaps the greatest force affecting healthcare. Conditions that often require surgery—atherosclerosis, degenerative joint disease, prostate disease, among others—increase in incidence with advancing age. With a few exceptions, it's time for all surgeons to consider themselves geriatric surgeons. Over 40% of surgeries in hospitals are done on seniors.

Several general principles can help guide surgeons who treat the elderly. First, the clinical presentation of surgical problems in the elderly may be subtle or somewhat different from that of the general population. This may lead to delays in diagnosis. In appendicitis, for example, a classic presentation occurs in less than one-third of elderly patients, resulting in perforation of the appendix, a serious complication, in over half of patients before surgery. Second, the elderly handle normal stress satisfactorily but handle severe stress poorly because of lack of organ system reserve.

With proper planning, surgery for seniors can go well.

Optimal preparation before the surgery is essential. Hypovolemia (dehydration), high blood pressure, bronchitis, and severe anemia should be corrected beforehand. When there isn't enough time for adequate preparation, risk increases. The results of elective surgery in the elderly are good in many centers. Results of emergency surgery are poorer but better than nonoperative treatment for most conditions. Therefore, it's often better to take care of a problem that could be treated electively, such as a hernia, rather than risk it leading to the need for an emergency surgery, when the risk is much higher.

Dr. Katlic has operated on numerous patients more than 80, 90, and even 100 years old, and these patients have done well. His team pays careful attention to details before, during, and after any procedure. One key is taking the time to review the goals of care with the patient so that everyone has a reasonable expectation of what will follow.

Based on his experience, Katlic maintains that

> ageism should be a thing of the past. A patient's age should be treated as a scientific fact and not with prejudice. Results of studies assessing surgery outcomes among the elderly do not support prejudices based on age alone. No particular chronologic age, of itself, should be viewed as a contraindication to surgery. Even an 80-year-old man is projected to have a life expectancy of 8 years. If such a person is in need of a lung cancer resection, he should be offered it because no other treatment is likely to give him those 8 years. Unfortunately, prejudice based on chronologic age (ageism) exists in both society and in medicine. In many cases, cardiac surgery may not even be discussed as an option for octogenarians with mitral valve disease, even though they could do well and get years of functional life. Studies also indicate that elderly patients with cancer are more likely to experience suboptimal staging and less aggressive treatment.

You may be surprised (as I was) to learn that people who harbor negative stereotypes of the elderly not only are unfairly biased against seniors but also put themselves at risk of ill health. This correlation was shown in studies by Professor Becca Levy of the Yale School of Public Health. She reported that people with ageism bias were more likely to develop Alzheimer's dementia themselves, noting that "we believe it is the stress generated by the negative beliefs about aging that individuals sometimes internalize from society that can result in pathological brain changes."

In the final analysis, making these decisions about surgery is complex for a variety of reasons, including physiologic variability among older patients. Therefore, each case should be evaluated on an individual basis. In the coming years, the number of elderly patients will increase dramatically, yet new surgical techniques are advancing as well.

Dr. Katlic sets out what needs to happen next: "We must put greater emphasis on optimizing outcomes for geriatric individuals, and it's paramount that all surgeons work hard to become better geriatric surgeons. In turn, we'll become better surgeons for patients of all ages."

CHOOSING HELPS MAKE HAPPEN
WHAT YOU WANT TO HAPPEN

As you could see in Alberta Cole's case (chapter 1), failure to make her wishes known led to all sorts of medical interventions. Whether these helped or hurt; whether she would have wanted them or not; whether the extra months of life battling bedsores, bladder infections, broken ribs, and dementia justified the pain she endured; and whether the expense was warranted are all questions that can never be answered. Nor could her family or doctors confidently make those decisions for her, especially when there was a difference of opinion among her children.

On the other hand, Michael and Joseph made their wishes known. Do you agree with their choices? Is this what you would have wanted for yourself? The power of the advance directive is that you can specify, in great detail if desired, what you would want and when. The advance directive is a living document (figure 3.1). Update it every 2 years or so, or whenever a significant change happens in your life: marriage, divorce, illness, matured children, financial loss or gain, or a move.

Figure 3.1. Outline of advance directive choices

What kind of care do I want?	Everything. Full-court press to the end.
	The middle path. As long as I'm functioning reasonably well, seem to be enjoying life, and am pain free, please keep me going with reasonable medical care.
	Don't do anything extensive or involved. Let nature take its course, and don't prolong the end.
Whom do I want to make decisions for me if I can't? And in what order?	__ Spouse or partner
	__ Adult child or children
	__ Parent(s)
	__ Sibling(s)
	__ Grandparent(s)
	__ Other family member: _____
	__ Friend
	__ Neighbor
	__ Combination of these: _____
Before making key decisions, my health care agent(s) should consult with	My doctor
	My best friend
	My spiritual advisor
	Other: _____
	Whomever they wish
	Combination of these: _____
	No one
Is there anyone I do not want to be involved?	Enter name here: _____

Figure 3.1 (*cont.*)

What do I want to be done with my body after I die?	Natural burial
	Conventional funeral and burial
	Whole body donation
	Consistent with my religion:
	_____
	Cremation and burial or scattering of ashes
How much do I want spent on the disposition of my body?	As little as possible
	A moderate amount
	Conventional funeral, casket, and headstone
	Whatever my family can comfortably afford
Do I want to donate my organs?	Yes, whichever organs will help others
	Yes, limited to the following: _____
	No

4

Cure vs. Healing

PALLIATIVE CARE AND HOSPICE

A dying man needs to die, as a sleepy man needs to sleep, and there comes a time when it is wrong, as well as useless, to resist.
—STEWART ALSOP

PALLIATIVE MEDICINE, OR SUPPORTIVE CARE

Palliative medicine and hospice care are two medical services that come up in any conversation about end-of-life care. Sometimes the terms are used interchangeably, but they are not the same. The confusion comes in part because patients may receive hospice care or palliative care, or both (table 4.1).

The National Hospice and Palliative Care Organization (nhpco .org) provides the following definition: "Palliative care is patient- and family-centered care that optimizes quality of life by anticipating, preventing, and treating suffering. Palliative care throughout the continuum of illness involves addressing physical, intellectual, emotional, social, and spiritual needs and facilitating patient autonomy, access to information, and choice."

What this means in practice is that a patient suffering from a serious illness will have not only a medical team focusing on a cure

Table 4.1. Palliative and hospice care: similarities and differences

Palliative care	Hospice care	What they both provide
Patient has any serious disease; best initiated at diagnosis of illness	Patient must have a diagnosis of a terminal illness	Supportive care for symptoms
Patient may be in any stage of disease	Patient must be deemed to have only 6 months left of life	Treatment for pain; provisions for comfort
May be fully or partially covered by insurance	Covered by Medicare, Medicaid, or private insurance	Family support and counseling
Compatible with and supportive of curative treatments	Does not provide curative treatments	Multidisciplinary care team
Usually initiated in the hospital and continued at home or other facility	Care is given at home, nursing home, or dedicated inpatient facility	Coordination with regular care team; patient and family are kept fully informed
Goal: to improve quality of life and coordinate care	Goal: to live in peace, comfort, and dignity until the moment of death	Valued services to patients and families in a difficult situation

but also a team focusing on symptoms, pain, and quality of life. Until recently, a palliative care consultation was usually requested only when all hope for cure was gone and no further standard treatment options were available. This request was often associated with the feeling of "giving up," and patients sometimes sensed that their doctor's focus had shifted away to patients who could still be helped. "Nothing more left to do, so let's send them to palliative or hospice care" is something I remember one colleague saying about a patient who was dying of end-stage heart disease. Or put colloquially: "Let's throw in the towel here. We're done."

Because of the historical—and unfair—negative connotations associated with palliative care, some institutions are now calling it "supportive care." That's certainly an accurate and probably a better description, but for now I will use the term "palliative" because it's more common. Palliative care is delivered by a multidisciplinary team with a variety of practitioners. Typically, this team includes doctors, nurses, pharmacists, and social workers, and often physical therapists, occupational therapists, dieticians, and pain management experts will contribute. Acupuncture, music therapy, and other complementary measures may also be included in the care. Palliative care can be provided in any setting: home, hospital, or nursing or rehabilitation facility.

Many nurses and physicians, including me, have come to believe that palliative care should be considered a regular and routine part of all medical care, from minor to the most severe problems. Often palliative care is employed at the end of life, but sometimes it is used in treating an illness that may last for years, such as multiple sclerosis. Palliative care should begin when the diagnosis is made. Hospice care, on the other hand, officially starts when there's a reasonable expectation that the patient will die within 6 months, although as you'll see in the next section, contacting a hospice before then can be worthwhile.

Although it might not be called palliative care (though it could be), the same principle of attending to a patient's symptoms and quality of life also applies in less extreme situations. Whenever I set a broken arm in the emergency room, I prescribe pain medication and suggestions for how to get through daily living with one's arm in a cast. The pain relief and care suggestions don't directly affect the speed with which the bone will knit back together, but we all know how important a person's comfort and peace of mind are to their healing and overall health. That's palliative care too.

In terms of serious illnesses, where the specialty of palliative care is making great contributions, we are beginning to see benefits beyond what anyone might have predicted. A *New England Jour-*

nal of *Medicine* article titled "Early Palliative Care for Patients with Metastatic Non-Small-Cell Lung Cancer" appeared in August 2010. "Metastatic" refers to cancer that has spread throughout the body, and "non-small-cell" is a type of lung cancer, one of the worst kinds and always fatal. In this study, palliative care was introduced early into the medical care plan. The results were surprising: "Early palliative care led to significant improvements in both quality of life and mood. As compared to patients receiving standard care, patients receiving early palliative care had less aggressive care at the end of life but longer survival." Furthermore, the "timely introduction of palliative care may serve to mitigate unnecessary and burdensome personal and society costs." In other words, the patients who received palliative care lived longer (about 2.7 months longer on average), were less depressed and/or happier, and the program saved everyone money. Let's see: people lived longer, were better off, and for less money. Sounds pretty good to me.

Palliative care leads to better outcomes and lower health care costs.

From a strictly scientific point of view, we can only speculate about the reasons why patients in this study lived longer. I believe it happened because the mind and body are interconnected at every level, although the mechanisms for this are not fully understood or appreciated. Perhaps living with less pain allows one's immune system to fight cancer better. Or maybe organs that would otherwise give out (heart, lungs, liver, kidneys), and whose failure leads directly to death, function more effectively when other symptoms and stresses are eased. Or maybe patients who are not in pain just eat better, thereby providing their bodies with nutrients that keep them going longer.

In any case, the implications are clear. Palliative care should not be considered after "everything else has been tried." Rather, it should be routinely included early for patients with serious short-term or long-term illnesses. As Dr. Steven Pantilat, professor of palliative care at the University of California San Francisco, put it, "If palliative care were a prescription, then every doctor would write it and every patient would want it."

Modern medical care can help cure disease. It can also help ease pain and suffering and improve patients' quality of life. We now know that these two objectives are fundamentally intertwined in our quest for longer and healthier lives.

Therefore, when you are completing your advance directive, you might want to include a statement that says, "Please provide me with palliative care at the earliest possible time, and please continue it for as long as necessary to help me."

Is it a doctor's job to cure disease? Or is it to heal patients? Curing means completely solving the cause of the problem. That can range from fixing a broken bone to eliminating the cause of an infection. Healing denotes making whole. What this means for medical practice is treating patients holistically by addressing their comfort, pain control, emotional state, financial condition, and family situation. Healing is a process; it doesn't always mean a person is cured but rather is supported in coping with all aspects of their medical situation. Curing may or may not include healing and vice versa. It's best when both goals are met.

HOSPICE CARE: I SHOULD HAVE CALLED SOONER

Because I could not stop for Death, he kindly stopped for me—
the carriage held but just Ourselves—and Immortality.
—EMILY DICKINSON

"I wish I had called hospice sooner" is the most frequent comment I hear about hospice. Hospice provides many benefits. I recommend that you start contacting and interviewing local hospices when the first "bad" diagnosis is made, even if you are several years from actually needing hospice services. Don't wait until the last weeks before death. You don't want to rush this decision when the end is near. If you do that, you will not get many of the services to which you are entitled. Like many big decisions, this one is best made when you are clearheaded and calm and not under pressure or in a time crunch.

If you are wondering whether it's time to call hospice, stop wondering. It's time.

We tend to think of hospice as providing only bedside care when the end is near. But hospice is not all doom and gloom. It's about making the most of the end of your life. It's about living life to the fullest and having the best end possible.

The National Institutes of Health describe hospice care as "end-of-life care provided by health professionals and volunteers." Hospice provides medical, psychological, and spiritual support. The goal of the care is to help people who are dying have peace, comfort, and dignity. Hospice employs palliative care as one of its tools, and its caregivers try to control pain and other symptoms so a person can remain as alert and comfortable as possible. Hospice programs also provide services to support a patient's family.

Hospice is a concept of personalized medical care specifically for those at the end of life when cures are no longer possible. It neither hastens nor postpones death. Rather it affirms life and regards dying as a normal process.

By Medicare's definition, hospice refers to patients whose life expectancy is less than 6 months. But too many people contact hospice too late in the process. The average service time in which hospice is involved with patients is just 2 months, and 40% are in hospice less than 14 days. This means that many people are missing months of service that could be of great benefit and to which they are entitled.

The concept of hospice is not new. It became established in England in the 1950s. Since then, hospice has grown to more than 4,000 separate programs in the United States. Some are freestanding; others are affiliated with other medical organizations, such as hospitals. Today more than 1.5 million Americans seek hospice service each year, and it is increasingly being recognized as an integral part of the health care delivery system.

Like the palliative care team, a hospice team includes practitioners from different fields, organized to meet each patient's individual needs. Hospice care can be delivered in a variety of settings, most often in the patient's home. Initially the team meets with the patient and family to assess their wishes, needs, and resources. Hospice workers come to the patient's home to provide care, including education for family members, pain medication, nutrition, and counseling. Other important support services may be delivered as well, including medical supplies, special foods, equipment, and respite care for home caregivers. Volunteers and other practitioners may provide services as diverse as music therapy, reading aloud, running errands, or pet care, depending on a patient's needs.

Hospice care can also be provided in hospitals, nursing homes, and dedicated hospice facilities. Regardless of the setting, the goal is the same: to provide dying patients with compassionate end-of-life care, to relieve pain and suffering, to offer support for family members, and to do so with respect for all concerned.

It takes a special person to choose hospice as a career. So often medical practitioners are trained to focus on "the cure," and sometimes we can enable that. But when cures are no longer possible, some practitioners feel they have nothing more to offer. That doesn't have to be the case, and that's where hospice comes in.

I've witnessed hospice personnel at work and was most impressed with their patience: how they took time to explain as much as possible about the dying process. Often patients don't fear death; we all know it's coming. But we do fear dying. Will we suffer? Will we be helpless? Will we have our loved ones with us? Hospice has many excellent resources about what to expect when someone is dying. Even family members who are not primary caregivers can benefit from these.

Modern hospice care offers reassurance that the dying process will be managed as comfortably as possible. Sometimes this means having a frank conversation about fears. Family members are taught when to call for an ambulance and when not to. Training is offered in daily care tasks such as bathing, dressing, and feeding. Pain medicines are used responsibly, as are sedatives and tranquilizers. It's not all about medicine: hospice brings a perspective on death and bereavement as a natural part of life's course.

Of course, like any service, hospices vary in their quality. Hospice is going to be part of your life for weeks or months, so it's a good idea to investigate hospices beforehand, whether for yourself or someone else. Be sure that all your questions are asked and answered. If you have special concerns, be sure these are addressed. If you can, try to meet some of the staff who might be providing care to you or your family member. That way, if any of the persons are not agreeable to you, you can ask the hospice to recommend others.

Medicare provides a website where hospice services are rated by customer feedback: www.medicare.gov/hospicecompare. There are both nonprofit and for-profit hospices, and you should make that determination as well. Personally, I prefer nonprofit ones as they generally are more concerned with patient care than profit. Another aspect to ask about is bereavement support. That is, what services, if any, are provided to the family after the patient dies. This can vary. Some might offer very little, maybe a monthly group meeting. Others might offer more substantial support, including individual or family counseling.

In your investigations of hospice providers, and for any serious medical discussion, it's a good idea to have someone else with you. When we are stressed, we tend to forget or misinterpret things. Having another person there can be helpful.

Too often people feel guilty or ashamed of their normal feelings of sadness or fear or even relief. Sometimes all a patient or family member wants is the chance to talk and be heard without worrying that the conversation will scare everyone away. Hospice care is sometimes seen as something outside the normal services of modern medical care, something to turn to when you've given up hope. Actually, hospice provides hope: hope that the transition from this world to the next will be made utilizing all the tools modern medicine can offer; hope that the end of life will happen with comfort and dignity; hope that suffering will be eased. Gradually, hospice is becoming accepted as a normal part of the health care sequence. In some communities, more than 60% of people use a hospice service, but in others, only about 20% do. One task before us is to make hospice readily available to all who need it.

To qualify for hospice benefits in the United States, a person must have Medicare Part A (over age 65) and be certified as being terminally ill by a physician, which means having a prognosis of less than 6 months to live if the disease runs its normal course. Benefits also allow for a one-time pre-hospice evaluation that could include a discussion of care options, pain management, and advance care planning. For adults younger than 65, private insurance usually covers these services at the Medicare rate. Children are generally covered under commercial insurance or Medicaid and under the provisions of the 2010 Affordable Care Act known as "concurrent care." Concurrent care allows pediatric patients to receive their hospice benefit along with curative treatment for their terminal diagnosis. For those without insurance, there are nonprofit hospices that will provide care as part of their charity mission.

Many hospices will provide services before the final 6 months begin. This would take the form of palliative care, and it would also give you an opportunity to get to know your hospice in advance. It's a "softer landing" when final hospice services are needed. Hospices can also help as care navigators.

Some hospices specialize, for example, by focusing on veterans and providing programs specifically for them. Some are able to help families with dying children, a particularly challenging service, but one that is certainly needed for these difficult situations.

Hospices sometimes help fulfill patients' final wishes. One hospice helped a 75-year-old man who was dying but not yet infirm; he had always wanted to skydive, and his hospice helped coordinate a jump. Another hospice supported a young boy dying of cancer who had anticipated having a military career; the hospice helped him get recognized by the local army base.

Again, the key point is this: contact hospice early, even before you need its services.

SPIRITUAL NEEDS

Lovers of truth—rise up! Let us go toward heaven.
We've seen enough of this world; it's time to see another.
—RUMI

Fortunately, our country enjoys religious freedom, and Americans have a wide range of beliefs and practices, whether religious or secular. Many people seek comfort and direction within the tenets of their belief system. The major religions have defined practices and customs for managing end-of-life care, and some have designed their own versions of an advance directive consistent with their beliefs.

A useful resource in the hospital is the pastoral care program. Chaplains may belong to different denominations, but they are trained to take care of people, upon request, from all backgrounds. In many hospitals, chaplains are also part of the hospital's end-of-life care team and patient care advisory board, which meet to review particularly challenging cases. Pastoral care programs also provide other services, such as therapeutic music for patients of all ages and conditions.

I've always appreciated the chaplains at the hospitals where I've worked. Not only do they help patients and families; they are there to support staff as well. It's nice when they come by to say hello and break up the stress of a difficult shift.

WHAT DOCTORS WANT FOR THEMSELVES

The most exquisite pleasure in the practice of medicine comes from nudging a layman in the direction of terror, then bringing him back to safety again.
—KURT VONNEGUT, GOD BLESS YOU, MR. ROSEWATER

As physicians, and for other health professionals as well, we are taught to "do no harm" and to do all we can for our patients. Traditionally this means giving patients every diagnostic test and therapeutic option to prolong life, even if sometimes this may lead to a worse quality of life. I've known doctors who kept their patients alive long past any hope of recovery. Doctors know how to present information in such a way that patients are moved toward decisions that the doctors favor. Please don't get the wrong idea. Most often this is done with the patient's best interests at heart. But doctors are human too, and these episodes bring up—consciously or unconsciously—our own anxieties about death and dying.

Nonetheless, when it comes to their own end-of-life care, physicians often anticipate an outcome for themselves that is different from what they recommend for their patients. We physicians have witnessed the dying process. While we may push patients into heroic lifesaving measures, we tend to choose dying at home for ourselves.

In personal conversations I have had with many of my medical colleagues (including physicians, nurses, physician assistants, pharmacists, paramedics, and others), many have shared with me that when they see the end coming, they'll have a plan. That plan could include squirreling away meds to relieve pain or even to hasten dying. We know the medicines, and we know what works.

Physicians have the power to write prescriptions and know how to space them out so that anyone reviewing prescribing habits would not detect a pattern. These prescriptions don't have to be for opioids, sedatives, or obviously toxic drugs. There are other medicines that can bring on or hasten death.

Some even have made specific arrangements with a spouse or other trusted loved one. In effect, they say, "When the end is clearly inevitable and there's absolutely no hope left and my quality of life is horrible, I trust you to make the right decision for me. That could include giving me the following medicines to ease my transition to death."

These plans also focus on what to do if dementia sets in. Clinicians have seen what happens when people become significantly demented. It's not pretty. There's no way to know what the life experience is for a person with dementia, but when you've seen enough of dementia up close, many clinicians say, "I don't want that for myself. I don't want to be fed, washed, dressed, and propped up in front a TV all day. I don't want to be drooling or doing embarrassing things like taking off my clothes, wandering about and getting lost, or attacking people close to me. I've seen Alzheimer's patients do that, and that's not how I want to end up."

Physicians' wishes for their own end-of-life care have been revealed in a series of studies. The most cited one was done in 2014 and published in the medical journal of the Public Library of Science. More than 1,000 physicians were surveyed, and over 88% said they would not want CPR in an end-of-life situation. That is, they would choose a DNR status. Furthermore, about 80% said that they would not want intense medical intervention if there were no hope of recovery.

Most significantly, the study concludes, "Our data show that doctors have a striking personal preference to forgo high-intensity care for themselves at the end-of-life and prefer to die gently and naturally. This study raises questions about why doctors provide care to their patients, which is very different from what they choose for themselves, and also [from] what seriously ill patients want."

These findings raise important questions: Why is there this disconnect? Why wouldn't doctors offer to patients what they want for themselves and their loved ones? Do they fear going against cultural norms? Are they concerned about a lawsuit or being reported to a medical licensing board for not providing proper care? Maybe we doctors fail to be totally honest with our patients.

Ask your doctor, Is this what you'd want for yourself?

When I am a patient or am talking to a doctor on behalf of a family member or friend about a test or a procedure, I ask, "If you were in this situation, or if it were someone you love, would you have this [test or procedure] done?" I've observed that this is a helpful question, and sometimes the doctor's whole approach changes.

No matter how I try to view this, I find this disconnect unsettling. We clinicians ought to offer our patients the best care we can. When discussing care options, whether in relation to end-of-life care or any procedure, our focus should not be on giving the most care or the least care possible but rather on the kind of care that's right for each patient. We have to end the disconnect between what doctors want for themselves and what we offer to patients.

> We come unbidden into this life, and if we are lucky we find a purpose beyond starvation, misery, and early death which, lest we forget, is the common lot. I grew up and I found my purpose and it was to become a physician. My intent wasn't to save the world as much as to heal myself. Few doctors will admit this, certainly not young ones, but subconsciously, in entering the profession, we must believe that ministering to others will heal our woundedness. And it can. But it can also deepen the wound.
> —ABRAHAM VERGHESE, CUTTING FOR STONE

5

Whom Do You Trust?

CHOOSING YOUR HEALTH CARE AGENT

———

I sustain myself with the love of family.
—Maya Angelou

THE STORY OF DAVE AND JACKIE STEVENSON

Dave Stevenson was 72 years old and had been in excellent health when he suddenly developed a severe headache, followed by slurred speech and paralysis of his left arm and leg.

Dave was a businessman. He owned a small liquor store specializing in craft beers. His daughter, Janelle, had taken over the enterprise and ran it on a day-to-day basis, but Dave still enjoyed coming to the store. He would show up 2 or 3 days a week. Many of the customers were regulars, and Dave liked socializing with them. His other child, Frank, had moved to Washington, DC, where he worked with the federal government.

Dave's wife, Jackie, was also an active businessperson. She ran a real estate firm. At age 70, she managed the office and handled some sales calls and open houses, although she left most of those tasks to the younger sales force. Jackie had years of experience and valuable tips on how to close deals.

Both Jackie and Dave were active in their community, particularly with their local Urban League's program for mentoring young people who wanted to learn more about business.

Dave was upstairs in the bathroom early Saturday morning when the symptoms struck. Jackie was downstairs, but she heard Dave groan and then slump to the floor. She ran upstairs and found him. With difficulty Jackie helped Dave move to the bed. He was conscious, though frightened, and he could still move one side of his body. Jackie called 911, then called Frank and Janelle, and waited for the paramedics.

While Jackie anxiously waited the few minutes for the paramedics to arrive, Dave's condition appeared unchanged. When they got there, the paramedics started an IV, applied a cardiac monitor, and checked Dave's blood sugar, all while getting a brief medical history. Sometimes low blood sugar can mimic a stroke, and if that's the case, the symptoms can be reversed quickly with intravenous glucose. But Dave was not a diabetic, and his sugar level was normal. So was his heart rhythm. The paramedics brought in a stretcher and called the hospital. They informed the emergency room nurse and doctor that they were bringing in a possible stroke victim.

"Stroke" is a general term that means the brain isn't getting an adequate blood supply. The region of the brain thus deprived fails to control the part of the nervous system that it is responsible for. A stroke in the speech center will cause a loss of speech, while one in the area that controls leg movement will paralyze that limb.

Loss of blood supply can happen for several reasons. The most common is a blocked artery, usually due to atherosclerosis, in which fat and cholesterol build up in the artery wall. Like an old pipe, the artery gradually narrows so that flow is reduced to a trickle and then blocked altogether. But a stroke can also be due to bleeding inside the brain. A blood vessel can burst, both interrupting its blood delivery and causing swelling that cuts off the flow of other nearby vessels. Or a bit of blood clot or tissue from another part of the body, usually the heart, can break off and travel through vasculature until the channel becomes so narrow that it can't pass any farther. This is called an embolus, which blocks blood flow in the vessel. Even a brain tumor can look like a stroke when symptoms start. The pressure of the tumor mass can also limit blood flow to a part of the brain.

A patient with a stroke from any of these causes can look exactly the same to the ER doctor. While there may be differences in the patient's history and ER exam that suggest one cause or another, the best quick test to find out what's happening is to get a CAT scan of the head. The scan can show blocked blood flow, bleeding, or a tumor. Each of these has different treatments, and a timely diagnosis is critical. For example, a blood vessel blocked by a blood clot might be treated with medications that dissolve clots. However, it would be disastrous to give that medication to someone who's bleeding in the brain and needs clots to form to stop it.

When Dave got to the ER, the staff was ready, having been alerted by the paramedics. Blood was drawn, an intravenous line was established, and a neurologist was summoned. If Dave's stroke were the result of a blood clot (the most common scenario), a neurologist would be needed to manage the complex medical treatment that would ensue.

Dave's condition was changing for the worse. His level of consciousness was decreasing, and he was slipping into a coma. To protect his airway and keep him breathing, the ER doctor intubated him.

Dave was taken to the CAT scan room with Jackie and a nurse at his side. The CAT scan took 10 minutes, and the on-call radiologist only needed to glance at the image to see what was going on. He called the ER doctor: "Mr. Stevenson has a massive intracranial hemorrhage. The bleeding is causing herniation." What this means is that the bleeding was so substantial that it was compressing the entire brain. The increased pressure inside Dave's cranium was pushing parts of his brain past their normal boundaries and down into his spinal canal.

The ER doctor immediately notified the neurosurgeon on call, as well as Dave's regular family doctor. She also took Dave's family to a private room to review the situation with them. Just as this discussion began, the ER doctor was pulled from the room because Dave's condition took a sudden downturn. He had a small seizure, and then he began what's known as decerebrate posturing. Dave's arms and legs became rigidly extended, his back and head arched backward, and his toes pointed down. This was a very bad sign, indicating severe, irreversible brain damage.

It had only been one hour since Dave fell in the bedroom at his home.

The neurosurgeon arrived, having already reviewed the CAT scan. He and the ER doctor met with the family, and they described Dave's circumstances: "Mr. Stevenson has had a massive brain hemorrhage. The bleeding is deep inside the brain. The parts of his brain not directly injured have been under tremendous pressure from the expanding bleeding, and now they are impaired as well. It only takes a few minutes of oxygen deprivation to cause irreversible brain damage."

Jackie asked, "Can't you operate and stop the bleeding?"

The neurosurgeon answered, "Of course we can always operate, but this would be major surgery, and it's very unlikely he would survive. And even surgery will not restore him. It might keep him alive a few hours or a few days. Because he's in good health otherwise, he might survive for as much as a week. At this point he's breathing only because a ventilator is breathing for him. His heart is strong and will keep beating, but his brain is dead. We're sorry, but there's nothing we can do. I wish there were, but realistically there isn't. You need some time alone to think about this."

Jackie, Frank, and Janelle struggled to take it all in. The shock was tremendous. Only an hour ago Dave was planning his day, full of activities. Now he was on a stretcher, effectively dead, his mind gone, his body living on.

The family went to the patient care room to be with their husband and father. They could see with their own eyes that Dave's body wasn't working. The ventilator hummed, moving the air in and out of his lungs. They held his hand and spoke quietly of their love

Sometimes families have only minutes to make life and death decisions.

and affection. They asked the ER doctor and nurse what was next. Dave would stay in the ER 2 to 3 more hours until a hospital bed was ready, and they could stay with him. But the staff said that the family ought to discuss what they wanted or what they thought Dave would want. Jackie knew that she and Dave had completed advance directives years ago. They were at home in a file cabinet. Frank went there to get Dave's.

Jackie recalled that Dave had served in the army in Vietnam. He had seen death, and he had seen men with terrible head injuries. He'd seen men who'd lost their ability to function and to think. Dave thrived on his independence, and he'd often said that he never wanted to burden his family.

When Frank returned, they read Dave's advance directive. In it, he had written that he did not want to be kept alive if he had no chance of recovery or if he had no chance of conscious life. He would want pain relief, but he would choose to allow nature to take its course. He did not want to be kept alive indefinitely by artificial means. He had designated Jackie his health care agent.

The family discussed Dave's wishes and the circumstances he was in. They asked the ER doctor to return. What would happen if Dave were admitted and kept on a ventilator? "Our best guess," she responded, "is that he could live for weeks or months, possibly even years. He would require constant care: feeding through tubes, complete personal hygiene. But he will not awaken, he will not talk, and he will not be aware of what's going on."

What if the ventilator were stopped and the breathing tube pulled out? "He would likely stop breathing in a few minutes or hours. He would die, although sometimes patients like him may last longer. There is no way to know for sure."

But aren't there people who are in a coma for years and then wake up? "There have been a few recorded cases, but even then, the recovery was minimal and not to any level of reasonable function. These rare cases have also been in younger people who suffered other kinds of brain injury, not the massive bleeding that is happening with Mr. Stevenson, where just about all the neurons in the brain are seriously damaged or dead."

DAVE'S DECISION ABOUT ORGAN DONATION

Dave's advance directive also noted that he wanted to be an organ donor. A kidney transplant had saved a friend's child, and this had inspired Dave. The family wanted to honor Dave's wishes, and the local organ donation organization was contacted. A Living Legacy counselor came to the hospital and joined the family. Questions were asked and answered. Was Dave too old to donate? No, age was not a problem. Dave's organs and body were in excellent shape, and everything would be closely examined before any transplantations were done. Would there be a cost? No cost to the family. Could they find out how Dave's organs were used? Yes, but only in general. Later, if the recipient agreed, contact information could be exchanged.

Jackie, Frank, and Janelle notified their extended family: the grandkids who ranged in age from 7 to 16, close family friends, and relatives. Their minister was called and joined them at the hospital. Over the next few hours, the family grieved over what had befallen their loved one, but there were also lighter moments, recalling many aspects of Dave's life. Dave was never left alone, as family members went in and out of the room, keeping constant vigil. A few hours passed, and the central question remained: What would Dave want now?

Eventually Jackie was able to come to a decision. Her voice was firm. "Dave and I have had a wonderful life. We've done everything we could hope to do: family, career, travel, and time together. But we decided long ago that we would respect each other's wishes when the end was near. Now it's that time for Dave. I know what he would want. He told us, and he wrote it down. He would not want to go on like he is now. He'd want us to remember him as we knew him: father, friend, member of the community. Let's all say goodbye. Then, let's bring the ER doctor back and ask her to pull the tube out and keep Dave comfortable until the end."

Dave died a few hours later. His organs were collected, and his gift saved three lives. Because Dave had thought this through, Jackie was in charge, conflicts were avoided, and Dave's choices were respected.

> *To be trusted is a greater compliment than being loved.*
> —GEORGE MACDONALD

> *All happy families are alike; each unhappy family is unhappy in its own way.*
> —LEO TOLSTOY

> *Happiness is having a large, loving, caring, close-knit family in another city.*
> —GEORGE BURNS

SECOND PART OF AN ADVANCE DIRECTIVE

The second part of an advance directive requires the important decision of who will be in charge if and when you are unable to make care decisions for yourself. Remember: if you are awake and competent, you make your own decisions, with or without the advice of others. But if you are unable to for any reason—coma, dementia, or while under anesthesia—then someone else must be designated. The person chosen to act on your behalf when you cannot is termed a "medical power of attorney" or a "health care agent." If you become unable to make your own health care choices, this person will have the authority to make them for you.

Typically the person chosen is an immediate family member. Most people choose their spouse or an adult child. But you could also choose a partner, close friend, or neighbor. In fact, it can be anyone you wish. It's also important to designate one or two backup health care agents in case the first-choice person isn't available. The names and contact information for the primary health care agent and the backups will be filled in on the advance directive form.

If you haven't completed an advance directive, most state laws specify a succession sequence. It usually goes spouse, adult children, siblings, parents (if they are around), friend, neighbor, and court-appointed social worker or guardian.

Once you've decided who you'd like to be your health care agent, you'll need to have a conversation with that person. This is key and always best done when you are well. Don't wait until you are ill, when your thinking and that of your health care agent may be clouded by emotion and stress. You should outline your values and goals and make sure that person understands them.

MAKING YOUR ADVANCE DIRECTIVE WORK FOR YOU

You can be as creative as you like. For example, let's say you have three adult children and no spouse. You could designate all three and allow for a majority vote for any contested decisions. Or you could specify one as being in charge, but that person would need to consult with the other two.

Do you have a domineering or annoying member of your family? Many of us do, and that person may stress everyone else or try to take over any situation. Or that person may become so emotional as to divert everyone's attention. Here's what you can do. You can specify that that person is not to be involved in decision-making or not even allowed to be in the room when these discussions are taking place. You can write, "Do not let Cousin Fred be involved in any discussion or decision regarding my end-of-life care, and I instruct my designated heath care agents not to discuss any aspect of my care with him."

What can happen when no one is specified? Conflicts may erupt between family members. For example (and I've seen this plenty of times), when no one is specified and there is more than one adult child, the adult children may disagree. These conflicts can become explosive. Or what happens when two siblings want different treatments for their brother? When this occurs, emotions run high and conflicts can escalate. Sometimes questions of money and potential inheritance cloud the medical decision-making process. Families can and do end up in court.

A living will should be a guide for a health care agent. However, many medical decisions do not fall into easily recognizable categories. Should pneumonia be treated with antibiotics? Is an MRI really needed to evaluate a change in mental status? Is it time to discharge the patient from the hospital to a long-term care facility?

You can assign other rights to your health care agent. For example, one form requests that the health care agent be allowed to ride in the ambulance with the patient and be given full hospital and health care facility visiting rights. This would include reviewing the patient's medical record and other personal health information. You can also request that your health care agent consult with certain designated individuals before making key decisions.

My advance directive asks that my adult children, in a case where my spouse is not available, consult with my best friend from medical school because I value his advice. However, he is not to be formally involved in making the final decision.

Giving a health care agent your medical power of attorney does not grant them the authority to handle your finances. While a health care agent can be given that authority, it is not included within the scope of an advance directive. It is also important to note that a health care agent is not responsible for your medical expenses. Some people might be dissuaded from serving as a health care agent if they thought that would make them liable for paying the patient's medical bills.

When does a health care agent take over for the patient? This is also addressed in the forms. There are two instances that trigger the authority of medical power of attorney. In the first, your health care agent takes over when your physician deems you incompetent to make medical decisions. The second arises when the patient, while still competent, authorizes the health care agent to take charge. For example, this might be useful for a patient undergoing extensive surgery followed by a prolonged recovery period. The health care agent could make decisions while the patient is recovering but still weak.

A health care agent can also be given the power to authorize an autopsy, make anatomical gifts, and direct the disposition of the patient's remains. All of these can become important under certain circumstances.

Because Dave Stevenson had specified that Jackie be his health care agent, she was able to make tough decisions about his care. Jackie consulted with her family, but the final decisions were hers alone. She followed Dave's wishes about organ donation, even if she might have disagreed with them or wouldn't have chosen organ donation for herself.

Many families struggle with these decisions when the patient has left no directions. Often arguments break out, sometimes with tears and yelling, leaving emotional scars that last for years. The designation of a health care agent spares the family the heavy burden of making group decisions at an intense time. The patient's wishes are specified and respected, and this eases the stress for everyone. Here's a personal story that changed my perspective.

I HAD A LEARNING EXPERIENCE

I was working a 4:00 p.m. to midnight shift when the ambulance call came in. An 88-year-old woman was found collapsed at home. Upon arrival, it was clear she had suffered a massive stroke, much like Dave's, and this was confirmed by a CAT scan. Before that episode, she had been functioning well at home.

The calls went out, and her family began to trickle in. The staff moved them to a private waiting area, and I shuttled back and forth, bringing them updates as the evaluation continued, in between taking care of other patients.

As the family gathered, it was clear that tensions were rising. Old wounds, jealousies, and grudges were emerging in this stressful situation. Those who knew her best, were closest, and saw her regularly said, "Please let Grandma die in peace." But the ones who were more remote would look at me and say, sometimes in an almost threatening manner, "Doctor, you do everything for her." This is a common pattern of behavior, and doctors and nurses are used to it.

Finally everyone had arrived, and all the evaluations and consultations were in. This patient had a large intracranial bleed with no hope of recovery. When I returned to the room, all hell was breaking loose. People were screaming, crying, or just huddled quietly. Eventually everyone turned to me; it was time for the doctor to speak. Fortunately, this woman had completed an advance directive, and a copy had been given to me. It was clear: if she were in a state from which there was no hope of meaningful recovery, she did not want heroic efforts. I read the advance directive to the family, adding that this was like she was speaking to me. I was legally and honor bound to follow her wishes.

I told them I would return to the patient's room, disconnect the ventilator, and turn off the medicines that were keeping her heart beating and her blood pressure up. I invited them to come with me. You might think at this point that the situation would get worse. But the opposite happened. They all quieted down. The decision had been made for them. The burden was lifted.

This patient, whom I never spoke with, taught me so much about the benefits of having an advance directive.

We went to the room, and I turned everything off. The family gathered at the head of the bed, stroked her hair, whispered in her ears, said a few prayers. I stepped back and watched all this. What had been an explosive situation that could have shattered this family instead became a healing moment.

The woman died peacefully in an hour or so. Proceeding with medical care would have only led to a vegetative state, with perhaps a few days in the hospital and then a gradual deterioration in a nursing home until death finally came.

I never would get a chance to know this woman or talk with her, but she changed my life. Her action—her completion of an advance directive—was a gift to her family. We say that we love our family, but do we do all the things we can that will help them when we are not there? One significant way to show our love is to take care of the paperwork that will support them in times of stress.

MOLST/POLST: WHAT ARE THEY?

I have seen that the prognosis may not be the reality any more than the map is the territory or the blueprint the building.
—DR. RACHEL NAOMI REMEN

There is a new document now legal in more than half the states in the United States, and more states are considering it. It's called

MOLST or POLST. The "M" or "P" distinction refers to which medical professionals can work with you to complete the form as determined by state law. "P" refers to "physician," and it means that only physicians can complete the form. In some states, other health care professionals can complete these forms with the patient. In those cases, the "M" stands for "medical" and refers to others who could do this in addition to physicians: nurse practitioners or physician assistants. In both cases, the "OLST" stands for "orders for life-sustaining treatment."

So, what are these new forms MOLST/POLST?

Each state has its own version, but all are generally the same in concept, so you'd have to investigate how it works in your state. I expect that, in years to come, these forms will evolve and become standardized. In the meantime, it may be something for you to consider. And while these forms are different from advance directives, they complement them.

So what are MOLST/POLST? These are medical orders, written by a medical professional using medical terminology, which specify what kinds of tests and treatments a patient may want. The professional reviews the orders carefully before authorizing them and should discuss each option and its implications with the patient. The forms are voluntary for the patient, but in some situations (such as a person on dialysis or someone being transferred from a hospital to a nursing home), medical personnel are required by law to offer one to the patient. Ultimately, though, the form is voluntary and can be changed anytime as needed.

These forms are typically used with patients who have advanced serious and complex disease, often in the last years of life. They facilitate communication among providers who care for the patient at different locations, such as a nursing home patient who is taken somewhere for dialysis and who may need emergency ambulance care or hospitalization from time to time. The form is to be completed in the context of their specific illness.

MOLST/POLST include what is commonly known as a "do not resuscitate" (DNR) order. Many practitioners, including me, have had difficulties with this term in the past because it sounded like we should withhold treatment under all circumstances. MOLST/ POLST approach this in a different way. Rather than a blanket DNR order, the form provides options for patients to choose from. For example, there are several levels possible in the provision of cardiopulmonary resuscitation (CPR). The patient can choose no CPR under any circumstances, limited CPR with no intubation or artificial respiration, or full CPR with all services available.

Note that pre-hospital care providers—paramedics—will be looking for and following these orders first, followed by other providers who become involved later.

An advance directive is filled out by you, and it spells out your wishes in general terms. But there are many times when decisions become hard to make. For example, what if a person with severe dementia breaks a hip? Should the break be surgically repaired? Let's say that it is, but then the person gets pneumonia. Should that also be treated, and if so, how aggressively? Intravenous antibiotics could be prescribed, but what if a ventilator becomes needed? An advance directive can't anticipate all possible clinical eventualities, and your designated health care agent (assuming you can't make these decisions for yourself) may find these choices difficult. MOLST/POLST can help.

A MOLST/POLST form gets much more detailed, and your provider can add specific circumstances where a test or treatment would or would not be used. This is something you and your provider discuss in advance. Some states require that the patient (or agent) sign the MOLST/POLST form before it becomes official. And like any medical order, the provider must sign it as well.

Here are the key items that these forms typically address:

- CPR or not, and if so, to what degree

- Respiratory support, ranging from full intubation, to only oxygen therapy, to none

- Blood transfusions

- Transfer to a hospital and under what circumstances

- Medical work-up, including how much testing and what types of tests

- Antibiotics, and if so, whether by mouth or by injection

- Artificial delivery of fluids and nutrition, ranging from never, to a trial course to gauge effect, to full support indefinitely

- Dialysis, ranging from none, to a trial to see if the kidneys recover, to sustained dialysis

- Blank space for other comments

As you can see, these can be complicated decisions, and ones that need to be discussed thoroughly with your provider before the forms are completed. Doing so allows you to clarify what your wishes are.

The key benefit of the form is that it travels with you as part of your medical record. For example, the form is useful to ER doctors because the patients who have one often end up in the ER. MOLST/POLST let us physicians know exactly what we should and should not do. Too many times a person with serious illness shows up in an extreme state, and we want to do the right thing. The problem is that we just don't know what the right thing is. These forms, when used properly, get that information to us securely.

MOLST/POLST and advance directives work together to offer fuller instructions for what kinds of care a person would want during a terminal illness (table 5.1). If you want to know about

MOLST/POLST, see https://polst.org, and if you want to know whether your state has legalized this form, see https://polst.org /programs-in-your-state. If your state is not on this list, I suggest that you contact your state's governor, health secretary, and state legislature to encourage adoption. The web address for an example of a MOLST/POLST form can be found in the Resources section of this book.

Table 5.1. Differences between an advance directive and MOLST/POLST

Advance directives are legal forms.	MOLST/POLST are medical orders.
For healthy people 18 years or older.	For people who have a serious illness or who are older and frail and who wish to specify treatment choices.
This **is not a medical order.** It is completed by you, and its instructions should be followed by medical staff.	This **is a medical order** decided on by you and your medical provider. It is signed by your medical provider, and its instructions should be followed by medical staff.
You give general instructions about the health care you would like in the future. You choose someone to make medical decisions for you if you later become unable to decide for yourself.	You state what specific treatments you want and do not want. Emergency and other medical staff must follow these instructions.
You can fill out the form on your own.	You fill out the form with your doctor (or nurse practitioner or physician assistant in some states).
You can change it at any time on your own.	You and your medical provider can change your MOLST/POLST at any time.
You are responsible for adding a copy of it to your medical record and making it available to your health care agent.	The form becomes part of your medical record. This means that medical staff can access it when they need to.

Source: Modified from Oregon POLST, https://oregonpolst.org/advance-directives

A LEGISLATIVE STORY: MY GOOD BILL WAS A FLOP

It's not easy to bring up the topic of end-of-life care to anyone. But imagine trying to do it as a politician running for office.

Politicians like to be at happy events, like groundbreakings for new buildings, ribbon cuttings for a new school or road, or graduations where the audience is filled with beaming parents. Going out into the community to discuss death, the events leading up to death, and severe and critical illness and injury does not exactly warm people up. As a physician, I ran the risk of being called "Dr. Doom."

I'd run into folks in the supermarket or the gym or other public places. They'd sometimes ask, "Delegate Morhaim, what issues are you working on?" I'd respond with an attempt at humor, "Your death. The death of your loved ones. The death of everyone you know. And don't forget to vote for me in the next election."

There's a degree to which the public appreciated my discussions. It's an awkward and uncomfortable topic, but they were grateful that someone had brought it up. In every community meeting, there were always people present who had recently been (or were currently) enduring a health care crisis of their own or that of a family member. This gave them a chance to feel less alone. Many had appreciated it, decades ago, when Betty Ford shared her difficult experiences with alcoholism or breast cancer. She opened the door for others to share their stories as well. Her approach is what I try to model when I bring up end-of-life care and the importance of advance directives.

However, trying to get legislation passed was another story. Fortunately, I wasn't the first to go down this path. The core legislation creating advance directives in Maryland had been passed in the early 1990s before I was elected. The attorney general's office had developed advance directive forms, and the excellent staff attorney Jack Schwartz became a local and national leader in this.

But there was more work to be done. Despite all these efforts, only about 35% of Marylanders had completed advance directives, and the rate was much lower in minority communities.

Almost all of my end-of-life care and advance directive bills gave my legislative colleagues the heebie-jeebies. But eventually, with persistence, many ended up passing and changing the legislative landscape.

One of the toughest, which did not pass, was House Bill 231 in 2003. It struck me that many people came across the idea of advance directives for the first time after they had gotten married, maybe had their first child, maybe bought their first home, and had begun to accrue some assets. Someone probably suggested that it was time for estate planning and a trip to a lawyer to notarize a last will and testament. These measures addressed financial issues and childcare. At these same appointments with a lawyer, an advance directive would also be offered but was often presented as an afterthought, as if it were optional. Many estate planning attorneys shared with me that wills would get signed straightaway but that advance directives would go unsigned for months or years. But because they had assets, these clients at least had heard about advance directives and had the forms offered to them.

What about people who didn't have money? Every person has had some thoughts about the inevitability of death. But folks with limited assets didn't have a reason to go to an attorney to plan for their disposition. Consequently, they were not offered the same information that people with assets were getting. It seemed to me that they deserved to have access to and to benefit from an advance directive just like anyone else.

Many of these people received financial aid from the state or federal government, such as Medicaid and pharmacy assistance. Why not use that interaction as a place to present information about advance directives? In fact, because these people were getting the benefit of substantial tax dollars that were spent on end-of-life care, why not require them to complete an advance directive as a condition of eligibility? That seemed like a good idea to me.

So I drafted a bill that would require adult applicants for state medical aid to be given information about advance directives and then would require they complete that form or else confirm with their signature that they didn't want to complete it. You can't force people (rich or poor) to complete an advance directive, but at least they would be required to make a choice about it.

I realized that a bipartisan approach was needed, so I pulled together cosponsors from both parties. I thought that this bill would appeal to legislators as a way to inform and empower poor people who didn't otherwise get to have these discussions and also to spare unnecessary medical expenses, especially government-funded ones. I had no idea of the furor that was to follow.

My left-wing friends accused me of wanting to kill off poor people, limit their individual freedoms, and set up a barrier to benefits for which they were entitled. Some darkly hinted that this was a plot to secure organ donation from poor people. Never mind that in my entire career as an ER doctor I had taken care of everyone regardless of their ability to pay and that as a legislator I had been a champion of better access to services for indigent populations.

From the right wing, my Catholic colleagues likewise got blowback, especially from the more intense "right-to-life" advocates. To them, this proposal was for nothing short of pulling the plug on people prematurely, a Dr. Kevorkian camel's nose under the tent, a slippery slope to euthanasia. Despite the fact that these otherwise conservative cosponsors had diligently opposed abortion rights, birth control, and Medicaid funding for abortions, they were directly challenged (and politically threatened) by these opponents of my drafted bill.

Our past records were disregarded by zealots. We got bashed from both sides by those who steadfastly refused to see the simple logic and benefits of this approach: giving people information about health care options, when they were in the process of applying for health care benefits, would lead to more personalized care for them (as wealthier people were able to arrange) while saving health care dollars for more productive use.

The end result is that the bill was significantly amended to create a task force to study increasing the use of advance directives. The bill passed the House of Delegates but died in the Senate. This effort was, in short, a flop.

The challenges I faced were not unique. My colleagues in other states had similar experiences, and no one can forget the bizarre and completely inaccurate argument about "death panels" that arose during the federal health care reform debate in 2009.

DEATH PANELS: SETTING THE RECORD STRAIGHT

Everyone is entitled to his own opinion, but not to his own facts.
—DANIEL PATRICK MOYNIHAN

Let's set the record straight about "death panels," a prominent controversy during the debate over the Affordable Care Act. This concerned how physicians could get reimbursed for taking the time—very important time—to have a conversation with a patient about end-of-life care. The then-current Medicare rules allowed for payment if the person was deemed to be in the last 6 months of life, and this guideline had been supported by both Democrats and Republicans. The change proposed in the Affordable Care Act would allow payment for this conversation between a physician and a Medicare patient to occur at any time, whether the patient was healthy or ill and as a part of routine medical care. This made perfect sense to me. These conversations are always better to have when there is no pressing medical issue on the horizon.

Former Alaska governor Sarah Palin coined the term "death panels," claiming that this new payment provision would empower government bureaucrats to decide which elderly persons would live and which would die. Some opponents of health care reform mistakenly (and creatively) argued that a section of the proposed law would create death panels and that government would be "pulling the plug on Granny." These panels would make similar judgments about other groups, such as those with Down syndrome, to determine whether they were worthy of receiving health care. Other prominent Republicans, including Newt Gingrich, Mike Huckabee, and John Boehner (then minority leader of the US House) picked up this argument as a way to undermine President Obama's proposed Affordable Care Act.

Death panels are made-up nonsense with no basis in fact.

There's a saying in legislative circles, "When in doubt, read the bill." So I actually read that section of the bill, and there was nothing in there about death panels or euthanasia. It was, as outlined above, a modest reform to a payment mechanism. What the legislation would do was, in fact, the opposite of what a so-called death panel would do. Without an advance directive, outside entities will make decisions for people. With an advance directive, individual rights are recognized.

Unfortunately, the media picked up on this catchphrase, broadcast it over and over again, and the death panel fiasco became part of the health care reform debate.

Worse yet, it actually worked. Not only did this reform not take place; some people became scared of having end-of-life discussions with their doctors. The chilling effect no doubt shut down some important health care conversations. But the fearmongering was without any basis in fact. It just confused people with made-up nonsense. It set back the discussion about end-of-life care, and—sadly—it succeeded in getting the funding for this important service struck from the bill, making it harder for physicians and patients to have serious conversations about end-of-life care.

Eventually, 7 years later, the payment reform originally suggested was adopted. Medicare now reimburses providers for having advance care planning discussions with patients regardless of their health care status. We can only wonder how many people in that 7-year period didn't get the care they needed because of this cynical political ploy.

A 2011 *Baltimore Sun* article about my efforts to promote advance directives summed up the matter well. Jay Hancock wrote that my goal was "individual responsibility, individual empowerment"; he added, "Humans are the only creatures that can contemplate their own demise. They might as well get ready for it. The best way to avoid an unwanted death panel is to set up your own."

6

It's Not Just about Old People

WHEN TRAGEDY STRIKES THE YOUNG

———

*Everybody has got to die, but I have always believed
an exception would be made in my case.*
—WILLIAM SAROYAN

WHEN THINGS GET TOUGH

Sometimes we have a negative magical belief system operating: if we think about something bad, it might come true. Of course, death will come true for us all eventually, but there's something inside us that thinks a discussion about death will bring it about sooner. No matter how we were raised or what our background is, we're all a bit superstitious on this point, and I'll admit to it myself. Eventually, I learned that having this discussion was not upsetting. The opposite happened. Talking about death brought me comfort, knowing that I'd taken important steps to be sure my wishes were recognized and that my family would not face conflicts, with the added burdens of guilt or anxiety, which could trouble them throughout their lives. Paradoxically, facing your fear of death can lead to a lessening of that fear. Making decisions about what you want changes a sense of helplessness into a feeling that you can exert significant control over what happens.

Let's see if we can break down some of the barriers. First, let's be up front and admit that this topic makes us uncomfortable. Then engage a trusted friend and discuss these issues in a private conversation. Small steps work well. Maybe scribble down some thoughts of your own. If you can, talk with people who lost a loved one a few years ago so that there's been time enough for them to reflect on those events. For some, it might be helpful to attend a Death Cafe (deathcafe.com) or similar event where people share perspectives and experiences about death. We all know that making important decisions can sometimes be hard, but most of us have learned that it can be done and that it's ultimately rewarding. First, let's review three famous cases that bear on this subject.

THREE FAMOUS CASES

Live as if you were to die tomorrow.
Learn as if you were to live forever.
—Mahatma Gandhi

We tend to think about end-of-life questions in the context of the elderly and the chronically ill, but the three most famous US legal cases on this issue all involved healthy young women. While most Americans are familiar with the case of Theresa Marie (Terri) Schiavo, whose "right to die" dominated headlines and caused national debate in 2004 and 2005, two landmark cases on this issue came much earlier. These three cases were all instrumental in changing attitudes, public opinion, and, ultimately, laws. As you read these tragic stories of family heartbreak, extensive medical treatments, and years-long legal wrangling, consider how the cases could be managed today if each of these unfortunate women had completed an advance directive. Their stories clearly demonstrate that advance directives are for everyone of adult age. Of course, how one completes an advance directive will change from age 18 to 28 to 58 to 88, which is why these documents need to be updated periodically.

KAREN ANN QUINLAN'S STORY

Over 40 years ago Karen Ann Quinlan was the center of what became the first major case on the complex legal issues around the right to die. The New Jersey Supreme Court characterized the case as a "matter of transcendent importance" because it raised two fundamental questions: (1) Is there a right to refuse lifesaving medical treatment? (2) And when, if ever, can a guardian exercise that right on behalf of an incompetent patient, meaning someone who is unable to make decisions for themselves?

Despite extensive testing, no cause was ever determined for 21-year-old Karen Ann Quinlan's collapse on April 15, 1975. Unable to breathe on her own, Karen was placed on a ventilator. As the months rolled by, she remained in a vegetative state with no higher brain activity. While the experts agreed that her chances for a return to any kind of functioning were remote, Karen Quinlan was not considered brain dead. As a result, her attending physicians, as well as the medical experts who testified at trial, concluded that to remove Karen from the ventilator would both deviate from the standard practice of medicine and be tantamount to a homicide and an act of euthanasia.

At that time, medical science was evolving so that patients who had previously died of conditions similar to Karen's were beginning to survive. But definitions of "brain death," "vegetative state," and "incompetent to make a decision" were still not well worked out.

At the beginning of the ordeal, Karen's parents authorized her treating physician to do everything in his power to keep their daughter alive, believing that she might recover. As their hope faded that Karen would regain mental functions, Mr. and Mrs. Quinlan sought the advice of their parish priest. He advised them that given Karen's circumstances, the termination of life support would be permissible according to the teachings of the Roman Catholic Church. The Quinlans asked the hospital to discontinue all extraordinary measures to keep Karen alive, including the use of a ventilator. They released the physicians and the hospital from any and all liability in connection with their actions. But even with the authorization and release, neither Karen's treating physician nor the hospital would agree to terminate the use of the ventilator.

Is there a constitutional right to die?

In 1975 it would have been highly unusual for a 21-year-old to provide any instruction to her parents and physicians in the event that she should become unable to manage her own care. Indeed, at that time very few legal and medical professionals had any concept of an advance directive or living will, and such documents were virtually unknown to individuals who were not involved in medicine or law.

Karen was quoted by her mother, her sister, and a friend as having made statements to the effect that she would never want to be kept alive by extraordinary means, in response to her having seen the deaths of family members and relatives of close friends. Mrs. Quinlan testified that Karen "was very full of life . . . and did not want to be kept alive in any way where she would not enjoy life to the fullest."

Given this evidence, Mr. Quinlan petitioned the New Jersey courts to appoint him legal guardian of Karen's person and property and to "intervene in the best interests of Karen Quinlan and allow her to die a natural death." The lower court ruled against Mr. Quinlan by holding that Karen's right to privacy, claimed by her father on her behalf, was trumped by both the medical professional's duty to provide life-sustaining treatment and the judicial obligation to choose continued life over death. Thus the court found no constitutional right to die that could be asserted by a parent for an incompetent adult child.

Mr. Quinlan appealed to the New Jersey Supreme Court. That court overturned the lower court's ruling and gave Mr. Quinlan the right to authorize the removal of the ventilator. It held that the constitutional right to privacy was broad enough to include an individual's decision to refuse medical treatment under certain circumstances. The court reasoned that if Karen had been able to make decisions for herself, she would have chosen to discontinue the use of the ventilator, even if that decision would result in her death. The court also said that Karen's individual rights had overcome the interest of the State of New Jersey, and thus she had a right to die.

The Quinlan court case was important for recognizing that the right to withdraw medical treatment is protected by the Constitution and that a designated guardian could make medical decisions for an incompetent patient. This was a remarkable shift away from the paternalism prevalent in the medical profession at the time, and it took a step forward in a trend toward patient autonomy.

The Quinlan case also recognized that the decision to withdraw life-sustaining treatment depends not only on whether a patient's existence may be prolonged but also on the quality of life the patient might reasonably expect. The Quinlans

Advances in medical care can raise complex legal and ethical issues.

won for their daughter the right to die "with grace and dignity," and she was weaned from the ventilator in March 1976. Karen continued to breathe on her own, and her parents chose to continue artificial feeding. Karen lived for 9 more years, until 1985, when she died at age 31 of respiratory failure brought on by pneumonia.

It was becoming clear that advances in medical care were raising complex issues. People could have their bodily functions sustained almost indefinitely, even if they couldn't think, move, or act for themselves. Who would make the decisions about their care, and on what basis would those decisions be made? *Quinlan* was the first major case to bring these issues to the fore.

NANCY CRUZAN'S STORY

Nancy Cruzan was 25 years old when, on the night of January 11, 1983, she was involved in a single-car accident in Jasper County, Missouri. Nancy had been thrown from her overturned vehicle and was found lying face-down in a ditch without detectable breathing or heartbeat. Although she never regained consciousness, paramedics at the scene were able to restart her breathing with a tube, and her heart began to beat again after stimulation with medication. At the hospital she was found to have severe brain injury, complicated by a long period without oxygen. Permanent brain damage results after 6 minutes of oxygen deprivation, and experts estimated that Nancy had been deprived of oxygen for a period of 12 to 14 minutes. Nancy remained in a coma, with no signs of higher brain function. Although she could breathe on her own, she could not swallow, so nutrition and hydration were provided by a gastrostomy feeding tube.

Despite intense therapy and rehabilitation over the following weeks, Nancy's condition did not improve. She was transferred from the rehabilitation facility to her home, where she was cared for by her family and round-the-clock nurses. After developing pneumonia, Nancy was admitted to Mt. Vernon State Hospital on October 19, 1983, where she remained in a persistent vegetative state.

Nancy's parents, Lester and Joyce Cruzan, had been appointed her co-guardians and conservators. In 1988, after four years with no improvement in their daughter's condition, the Cruzans asked the court for permission to stop artificial feeding and hydration.

At the trial, the court heard extensive testimony from physicians and nurses, and it concluded that Nancy had lost all higher brain functions, as well as the ability to swallow food and water, and that this condition was irreversible. The trial court further found that Nancy had said, in a conversation with her housemate, that she did not want to be kept alive by artificial means if she could not live "halfway normally." The court concluded that to deny Nancy's parents the authority to act under these circumstances would be to deprive Nancy of equal protection under the law. The court ordered the state hospital employees to carry out the wishes of Nancy's parents and withdraw her feeding tube. In part because this was a case without precedent, Nancy's court-appointed guardian appealed the decision.

The Missouri Supreme Court overturned the lower court by ruling that there was neither a constitutionally protected right to die nor sufficiently clear and convincing evidence that Nancy Cruzan would not wish to continue her vegetative existence. The majority further found that her parents, as guardians, had no right to make decisions on their daughter's behalf. Cruzan's parents appealed the Missouri decision, and in December 1989 the US Supreme Court heard its first case concerning the right to die.

The *Cruzan* decision overturned the previous *Quinlan* case in that the Supreme Court held, first of all, that any right to refuse treatment had to be balanced against a state's legitimate interest in maintaining life. Second, the majority of the justices rejected the idea that a person's quality of life should be considered in deciding whether to terminate life-sustaining treatment. Third, the court decided that statements made by Nancy Cruzan to her housemate did not meet the "clear and convincing" standard of proof required by Missouri law. However, Justice Sandra Day O'Connor, while voting with the majority, took a different approach. She made it clear that the court's decision was to be applied only to the Missouri statute. She wrote that "the Court does not today decide the issue whether a State must also give effect to the decisions of a surrogate decision-maker." This meant that other states would have to resolve the matter for themselves.

Justice O'Connor's opinion motivated both the federal and state governments to enact or clarify laws pertaining to living wills and advance directives. In 1991 the Patient Self-Determination Act was passed by Congress and signed into law by President George H. W. Bush. All 50 states and the District of Columbia followed with laws of their own.

Two months after the Supreme Court's decision was issued, Nancy's parents asked the state court to consider new evidence from several of their daughter's coworkers. The coworkers testified that Nancy had said she would not want to live "like a vegetable." The judge ruled that these statements provided clear and convincing evidence of Nancy's intentions and ordered the hospital to comply with the request of Nancy's parents to have her feeding tube removed. This was done on December 14, 1990, and Nancy Cruzan died 12 days later, at the age of 33, surrounded by her family—6 months after the Supreme Court's ruling and almost 8 years after the accident.

THERESA MARIE (TERRI) SCHIAVO'S STORY

The case of another young woman, Terri Schiavo, became a contentious issue in the debate over the right to die and the right to privacy. Ultimately the case involved advocacy groups on all sides, as well as the president, Congress, and even the Vatican. Six times over the course of the case, the US Supreme Court was asked to rule, and each time it declined to do so.

Terri Schiavo had been living in a persistent vegetative state since a cardiac arrest in 1990. In 1998, after many years of failed attempts to restore her brain function, Terri's husband Michael, as her guardian, asked that artificial feeding be stopped "so that she would die a natural death." He said that this was her stated preference should she ever become incapacitated with no hope of meaningful recovery. Terri's parents disagreed, arguing that their daughter was not in a persistent vegetative state and that, even if she were, she would not have wanted to have artificial life-support removed.

Beginning with a trial in the Florida courts, the issues were litigated, appealed, and litigated again. Terri's feeding tube was removed for the first time in 2001 but then was reinserted 2 days later, pending the outcome of an appeal by her parents. The appeal was rejected, and the tube was removed again in 2003. Within 6 days the Florida legislature and Governor Jeb Bush enacted "Terri's Law," mandating the tube's reinsertion. Subsequently, Terri's Law was declared unconstitutional by the courts, and on March 18, 2005, Terri Schiavo's feeding tube was removed for the third and final time.

In the meantime, a media frenzy had begun. The *Schiavo* case was the number-one topic on the 24-hour news cycle, on talk shows, and at kitchen tables around the country.

Two days later, on March 20, Congress passed emergency legislation (the "Palm Sunday Compromise") to allow Terri's parents to petition the federal courts for the feeding tube to be reinserted. President George W. Bush flew back to Washington, DC, from his vacation in Texas to sign the bill, and Terri's parents immediately followed up with a petition for an injunction in the federal district court. Arguments were heard the following day, after which the judge declined to order the reinsertion.

The next day, the Eleventh Circuit Court of Appeals in Atlanta upheld the federal district court's ruling, and one day later the US Supreme Court once again refused to hear the case. This effectively ended all further appeals. Terri Schiavo died on March 31, 2005, with Michael at her side. An autopsy revealed extensive and irreversible brain damage.

One thing was clear from the beginning: had Terri Schiavo completed an advance directive, her wishes—whatever they were—would have been known, and the firestorm of family, legal, and political conflict would have been avoided.

THIS IS IMPORTANT FOR YOUNG PEOPLE TOO

When your mother asks, "Do you want a piece of advice?"
it's a mere formality. It doesn't matter if you answer yes or no.
You're going to get it anyway.
—ERMA BOMBECK

The legal and medical circumstances of Quinlan, Cruzan, and Schiavo are relevant for all of us. Every time I speak publicly about the need for advance directives, I get a range of reactions from audience members. "Why do I need one of those? I'm in good health." "This is for grandma and grandpa, not me." "This makes me sad. I'd rather not think about it."

In some respects, it's more important for younger people to complete advance directives than for elders. They are generally in good health, and the life-and-death situations younger people confront tend to be sudden and catastrophic. Older people, on the other hand, usually get a bad diagnosis and have a few years to sort matters out. But younger people tend to get struck down in a bad accident or a major disease process, like leukemia, a drug overdose, or a subarachnoid hemorrhage (a burst blood vessel in the brain).

Older people usually have established relationships with people who know them well and can help with major life decisions, whereas younger people can still be exploring who and what are truly important to them.

I remember the first important time that my wife, Shelley, and I confronted this issue. We'd been married about 3 years, and we had just had our first child. We were considering buying a house. I was still in debt from medical school, but I landed my first regular job, and we were beginning to dig our way out into a more stable financial situation. It seemed time to make out a will. It dawned on us that we were now really adults. What if something were to happen to one of us, or worse to both of us? We needed a plan.

We contacted a lawyer and began the process. We didn't have too much money, so the financial part went quickly. We also decided whom we'd ask to raise our daughter if we weren't around, not an easy decision but one we had to make. Then came the last document in the package. It was the advance directive, and it struck us as unnecessary. We were young, in good health, so why was this needed? The advance directive sat there for a couple of years, incomplete. Of course, we eventually got around to completing it, driven by other life experiences and by common sense.

Many young people have the same reaction we had. Why bother? The answer, however, is simple. You just don't know what is going to happen to you or when. Like the Boy Scout motto: be prepared.

When our children turned 18, we gave them advance directives to complete. One pointed out that she'd made a decision about organ donation when she got her driver's license about a year before. A few years later, we had a family gathering. At that time, our adult children were living in New York, Los Angeles, and Boston, so I downloaded the advance directive forms from each state. We discussed the issues briefly; everyone completed their forms; and some neighbors came over to witness the signing. I copied the forms and emailed them so that we each had a copy of all of them. It was an easy process.

Advance directives are about being prepared, about taking steps to spare others unnecessary heartache. Everyone should complete one, and there's no excuse not to.

THE MEDICAL TEAM AND YOUR KEY QUESTIONS

Working with your medical team is key, and the best place to start is with your primary care doctor if you have one. Have the conversation about your advance directive and what you want. Ask your questions and get answers. It likely will take several visits to sort out your concerns and resolve them. Do this when you are healthy and not facing any problems. That's the importance of *advance* in the term "advance directive."

Here are some ways to start that conversation with your doctor:

- Doctor, I want to schedule a few minutes where we can sit down, uninterrupted, to talk about my end-of-life care wishes.

- I'm worried about my end-of-life care and want to complete an advance directive. Can you get me information about this?

- One of my concerns is that if this disease process continues, I'll be a burden to my family. What can I do about that?

- A friend of mine died recently, and it was a fraught process that I wish had been handled differently. How can I avoid that happening to me?

- I have strong beliefs about end-of-life care, and I want to be sure you are okay with these since I will be relying on you for medical care.

- What happens if I can't swallow food on my own?

- What is brain death, and how is that determined?

- What if I change my mind about what's in my advance directive?

Often, though, you won't get to choose your medical team. You or your loved one may be brought to an ER and treated by strangers who are busy and seem distracted. It can be a tough situation, but there are some things you can do. Tell the doctor or nurse, "I see you are very busy, but when you can take a few minutes, I'd like to discuss my loved one's care with you." Almost all hospitals have support staff. Their job title may be "care manager" or "social worker." These people can intervene for you.

All hospitals also have a pastoral care department with chaplains on staff. If not already there in the hospital, a chaplain can be called in to see you. Chaplains are well versed in hospital procedures and jargon, and they know the medical team. In many hospitals, chaplains participate in medical rounds in the intensive care unit along with nurses, doctors, pharmacists, and other specialists. They can intercede on your behalf and work with you to make sure your concerns are addressed. They can help with the completion of an advance directive if you have not done that already.

Personally, I've always enjoyed talking with my hospital's pastoral care staff. We providers get stressed too, and sometimes a friendly chat lowers my own tension levels. I've worked in hospitals with clergy of various religious affiliations (mainly Catholic, Protestant, and Jewish but also Navajo Indian and Muslim), who take care of people of all faiths and backgrounds (including agnostics and atheists). I've always found chaplains to be friendly and accessible. This group is a great resource and one that you ought to use, even if you are not a person of faith.

You may be familiar with the term "doula." It refers to someone who is not a health professional but is trained to support someone through a challenging time. Typically, doulas provide support in childbirth. In that situation, think of the doula as a coach and companion who is there to support the mother and her family and who works with the medical team as well. This support can come during pregnancy, labor and delivery, and also postpartum.

There are now end-of-life doulas as well, for that other universal human experience, death. End-of-life doulas are there to support people and families as they approach death. This support can come soon after a diagnosis, in the last days of a person's life, and in the time after death when the family needs support. Generally doulas are employed for deaths at home, but there is no reason that an end-of-life doula could not tend to someone who is dying in a hospice facility or hospital instead.

If it suits you, support can come from many sources, including pastoral staff and end-of-life doulas.

Hiring a doula is worth considering, as they can provide respite and support for other family caregivers as well. Doula services are not covered by insurance, so there will be a cost. If you are interested in this, you should evaluate the options early in your planning process. The doula will become an important part of your medical team.

NO ONE SHOULD DIE ALONE

Security is mostly a superstition. It does not exist in nature, nor do the children of men as a whole experience it. Avoiding danger is no safer in the long run than outright exposure. Life is either a daring adventure, or nothing.
—Helen Keller

There are people who want to be alone when they die. I've heard of some who choose to venture into nature toward the end of their chronic illness and die peacefully alone. Others get tired of having too many people around who are not providing comfort, and they may prefer to have just one or two close friends and family members as the end approaches. In the introduction I cited statistics showing that most Americans want to die at home with close friends and family nearby. But it may not always be possible to have that.

That is why a service called No One Dies Alone may be of interest. It was started by Sandra Clarke, a registered nurse, who has told her story of coming to work on a night shift. A very sick patient, with a DNR directive (do not resuscitate), asked her, "Will you stay with me?" Sandra had obligations to other patients and thought she'd return when she could. But when she did finally get back, the patient had died. Sandra felt "frustration and anger" that she could not help this man who had a "simple wish that could be easily granted." That motivated her to find a way to provide patients "some comfort at the end of life."

Inspired by that experience, she started No One Dies Alone, a nonprofit volunteer organization that serves people who might otherwise be alone at the end. Volunteers go through a training program first and then are on-call. Those who have volunteered say the experience is valuable for patients and for themselves as well.

Since the exact moment of death can't be predicted, volunteers spend 2 hours or so at a patient's bedside in shifts. Sometimes volunteers will stay at the bedside during a vigil to give family members a respite. No One Dies Alone providers tell us that the greatest fear dying patients have is not death or suffering with pain. The reality of a chronic illness somehow prepares them for death, and modern medicines can manage pain and anxiety. What they do fear is being alone and emotionally abandoned. Often, they just want human presence and touch. More and more hospitals and hospices are providing this service, and perhaps this is something you might seek out for yourself or even want to do for others.

7

No Easy Answers

DEMENTIA, THE SYSTEM, AND GETTING IT RIGHT

———

My grandmother started walking five miles a day when she was sixty.
She's ninety-seven now, and we don't know where the heck she is.
—ELLEN DEGENERES

THE DEMENTIA CHALLENGE

Even when all the best efforts are made and everything is done right, sometimes there are no easy answers.

Over half of all people who live past age 85 develop some form of dementia. It may be relatively mild and non-progressive, or it may be severe and progressive. All dementia is produced by some type of injury to the brain.

Whenever dementia is mentioned, people immediately think of Alzheimer's disease. It's the most common and well-known form of dementia, but there are other kinds and causes of dementia. The other common dementias are vascular, Lewy body, Parkinson's related, frontotemporal, Huntington's, Creutzfeldt-Jakob, normal pressure hydrocephalus, Wernicke-Korsakoff, syphilis, and Lyme disease. There are dozens of rarer ones, usually caused by a genetic condition.

The symptoms of these various diseases overlap and typically include memory loss, confusion, and emotional instability. Sometimes there are associated physical symptoms as well, such as trouble with walking.

For someone with symptoms of dementia, a comprehensive medical evaluation is essential. The medical team must first evaluate and rule out other significant medical conditions, such as brain infections, tumors, or blood clots in or around the brain (cerebral hematomas). After that first evaluation, more detailed testing is indicated because an accurate diagnosis directs treatment. Consultation with a physician specialist is needed to sort out these various dementias through a careful history and physical exam, along with lab and imaging tests. Too often, people with early dementia symptoms are told they have Alzheimer's without undergoing an adequate work-up.

In some cases, there are specific treatments. Hydrocephalus can be treated with a special tube that drains fluid from around the brain. Wernicke-Korsakoff is most common in alcoholics and in those with poor nutrition and can be treated with thiamine (vitamin B1). Syphilis and Lyme disease can be treated with antibiotics.

In the other cases, there are treatments that can slow the progress of the disease or ease its worst symptoms, but these treatments are only temporarily effective. Unfortunately, as of now, for most dementias there are no treatments that can cure or significantly alter their course. Hopefully, research will identify new treatments and also pin down the underlying causes of these dementias.

Alzheimer's disease, which results from brain degeneration, was first described in 1906 by the German physician Alois Alzheimer. While studying microscopic slides of brain tissue from deceased dementia patients, he noticed characteristic plaques and tangles among the nerve cells. Since the early twentieth century, the disease has become widely recognized and studied.

Alzheimer's disease can only be definitively detected by examining brain tissue. Therefore, a diagnosis of Alzheimer's cannot be confirmed without a brain biopsy, which is rarely performed on living patients. Generally it's found on autopsy. Because the constellation of symptoms is well established, and once the other possibilities are eliminated, Alzheimer's disease is then diagnosed as the likely candidate.

The cause of Alzheimer's is not known, although research has shown that certain lifestyle factors and treatable diseases can make a person more likely to develop this type of dementia. These risk factors include smoking, excessive alcohol consumption, diabetes, high cholesterol, high blood pressure, insulin resistance, obstructive sleep apnea, thyroid abnormalities, periodontal disease, high-fat diets, and vitamin B12 and vitamin D deficiencies.

Whatever the cause, there is no specific treatment, though there are useful care plans that can be developed on an individualized basis. Over 5 million Americans are currently living with Alzheimer's disease. By 2050 that number will rise to 13.5 million.

The economic impact of Alzheimer's and other dementias is staggering. Dementia affects the brain, but the body usually degenerates at a much slower rate, so it can take a long time until death arrives. During these years—or decades—as the dementia progresses, a patient with dementia needs increasing amounts of care.

RONALD REAGAN TELLS HIS STORY

Often the symptoms begin insidiously. Forgetting where you left the house keys is something that happens to everyone. But with the onset of dementia, these rare events start to happen more and more often. Eventually an affected person begins to lose track of things that are not normally forgotten, such as a friend's name or one's own street address or how to do a simple calculation. Sometimes mood changes are the first indicator of dementia. Early on the patient is aware of the symptoms. Former president Ronald Reagan wrote movingly about this in a letter to the American people:

I have recently been told that I am one of the millions of Americans who will be afflicted with Alzheimer's disease. Upon learning this news, Nancy and I had to decide whether as private citizens we would keep this a private matter or whether we would make this news known in a public way. In the past, Nancy suffered from breast cancer and I had my cancer surgeries. We found through our open disclosures we were able to raise public awareness. We were happy that as a result many more people underwent testing. They were treated in early stages and we were able to return to normal, healthy lives. So now, we feel it is important to share it with you. In opening our hearts, we hope this might promote greater awareness of this condition. Perhaps it will encourage a clearer understanding of the individuals and families who are affected by it. At the moment I feel just fine. I intend to live the remainder of the years God gives me on this earth doing the things I have always done. I will continue to share life's journey with my beloved Nancy and my family. I plan to enjoy the great outdoors and stay in touch with my friends and supporters. Unfortunately, as Alzheimer's disease progresses, the family often bears a heavy burden. I only wish there was some way I could spare Nancy from this painful experience. When the time comes, I am confident that with your help she will face it with faith and courage. In closing let me thank you, the American people, for giving me the great honor of allowing me to serve as your president. When the Lord calls me home, whenever that may be, I will leave with the greatest love for this country of ours and eternal optimism for its future. I now begin the journey that will lead me into the sunset of my life. I know that for America there will always be a bright dawn ahead. Thank you, my friends. May God always bless you.

Fortunately, President Reagan was able to afford the expensive individual care that helped keep him alive for years, while sparing his family many burdens.

For most Americans, though, dementia leads to great personal and economic hardship. It can cost many thousands of dollars each year to take care of a person with dementia. Dementia makes up the largest single principal diagnosis by percentage of Medicare payments for hospice care. This will only increase as more of the population ages and lives longer.

President Ronald Reagan revealed his diagnosis of Alzheimer's disease in a letter to the American people.

An advance directive can be customized to address dementia directly. A friend of mine forwarded to me an addendum to his advance directive that provides instructions for how he'd like to be treated should he develop advanced dementia. It's worth reviewing as an example of how this difficult situation can be managed and how an advance directive can be modified to reflect personal values and circumstances. There is no requirement that something like this be done. You could modify these instructions to suit your own wishes or not include such instructions at all.

Dementia Provision (Advance Directive Addendum)

I, _____, am creating this document because I want my health care representatives/agents/proxies, medical providers, family members, caregivers, long-term care providers, and other loved ones to know and honor my wishes regarding the types of care I want to receive if I develop an advanced stage of Alzheimer's disease or other incurable progressive dementia.

Under the conditions of advanced dementia, including my inability to communicate rationally with loved ones or caregivers, and/or my physical dependence on others for all aspects of bodily care, continuing life would have no value for me. In those circumstances, and if my condition is unlikely to improve, I would want to die peacefully and as quickly as legally possible to avoid a drawn-out, prolonged dying that would cause unnecessary suffering.

I request the following, as marked:

_____ To receive comfort care only, focused on relieving any suffering such as pain, shortness of breath, anxiety, or agitation. I would not want any care or treatments that would be likely to extend my life or prolong the dying process. This includes life-sustaining measures like cardiac pacing, cardiopulmonary resuscitation, and mechanical ventilation.

_____ In the event of any acute infection, I do not wish to be treated with antibiotics and/or antimicrobials in any form but treated only for aggressive pain and symptom relief, while the illness takes its natural course.

_____ If I lose the ability to speak for myself and my advance directive is being taken into consideration as written, I also would like it to be clear that if I am currently receiving any medications or treatments that are likely to extend my life or prolong my dying process, I would like those to be stopped.

_____ I request that food and fluids in any form, including spoon-feeding, be stopped if, because of dementia, any of the following conditions occur:

I appear indifferent to food and being fed.

I no longer appear to desire to eat or drink.

I do not voluntarily open my mouth to accept food without prompting.

I turn my head away or try to avoid being fed or given fluids.

I spit out food or fluids.

I cough, gag, choke on, or aspirate (inhale) food or fluids.

_____ If the above statement regarding food and fluids goes into effect for any of the above listed reasons, and as a result I begin to experience delirium, agitation, or hallucinations, then I would like my medical team to provide palliative sedation in order to alleviate my suffering until death occurs.

_____ I want the instructions in this dementia provision followed even if my caregiver or health care agent judges that my quality of life, in their opinion, is satisfactory and I appear to them to be comfortable. No matter what my condition appears to be, I do not want to be cajoled, harassed, or forced to eat or drink. I do not want the reflexive opening of my mouth to be interpreted as my giving consent to being fed or given fluids or interpreted as a desire for food or fluids. I have given considerable thought to this decision and want my wishes to be followed.

Before I am admitted to a long-term care facility, I want the facility to affirm its willingness to honor these instructions. If the facility where I already reside will not honor these instructions, I want to be transferred to one that will.

Printed Name: _____ Date of Birth: _____

Signature: _____ Date: _____

We, whose names are provided below, declare that the person who signed this document is personally known to us, appears to be of sound mind and acting of their own free will, and signed this document in our presence.

Witness 1 Signature: _____ Date: _____

Witness 2 Signature: _____ Date: _____

THE COSTS OF DEMENTIA

Some people plan ahead by purchasing long-term care insurance. This insurance can cover part of the cost of nursing home care, as well as home care. Premiums for such policies can run high, and their benefits vary, depending on the level of coverage purchased. As with other insurance, such as for your car or your home, it is impossible to predict if the coverage will ever be needed.

For people with substantial financial resources, a continuing care retirement community (CCRC) is another way to plan ahead. Such facilities attract seniors who enjoy both mental and physical health. Should the person later need extra care, they can move into the CCRC's assisted living facility or nursing care facility. Buying into a CCRC can cost anywhere from $60,000 to over $400,000, plus monthly fees that range from $1,000 to $6,000.

People without insurance or sizeable savings who have a catastrophic or long-term illness such as dementia are often forced to "spend down" virtually all their assets. For these people, a lifetime of accumulated funds is exhausted on health care. This system-imposed poverty eventually makes the person eligible for Medicaid, at which point health care costs will be paid for by the government. However, any provision for a spouse or any inheritance for children is gone. Some couples have been advised to file for divorce as soon as they learn one of them has Alzheimer's, in order to protect the healthy spouse's assets. You wouldn't think a situation could be made more heartbreaking than receiving a diagnosis of Alzheimer's disease, but under our current health care regime, it is entirely possible.

Beyond the financial expenditures, the human costs are immeasurable. At first, most Alzheimer's patients can be taken care of at home. But as the disease takes its toll, symptoms often become worse. Stresses on caretakers mount. A person who has Alzheimer's disease requires constant supervision, as well as help with the basics of daily living: feeding, getting dressed, bathing, and going to the bathroom. And as time goes by, that person's demands for attention grow. The patient may become incontinent and unable to climb stairs or swallow solid food. Care for the caretakers becomes more important, but respite from these demanding chores is often hard to arrange.

Eventually medical issues arise. These sometimes are related to the dementia (such as developing an infection because of poor hygiene), but more often they are caused by the many diseases that afflict elderly people. In those situations, caretakers have to make medical decisions for their loved one. These are often challenging. How can they tell what the patient is thinking and feeling? What is a person's inner life like when they can no longer speak? Are they happy or miserable? Do they have any awareness of what's going on? Is it time to make a move to a nursing home? When does "care" create more suffering than healing? More pain than comfort? For a loving spouse or adult child who has been designated the health care agent for a patient with Alzheimer's disease, these are difficult questions.

One such caregiver got a call in the middle of the night from a hospital's emergency department. His mother had fallen at the Alzheimer's disease facility (usually called a "memory care center") where she lived and was taken to the hospital by ambulance. At the ER, the son learned that his mother's hip was broken. Although she had lost her ability to speak some years before, it was clear that she was in pain, and the only definitive way to relieve that pain was with surgery. But surgery would also be an agonizing experience, and she didn't have enough mental ability left to carry out a rehabilitation program after surgery. She'd never walk again, with or without the operation. Her son gave the go-ahead for surgery. His mother's hip was pinned, and she made it through a difficult convalescence. Since physical therapy was impossible, her eventual recovery only allowed her to sit up for a few minutes each day. Otherwise, she was bedridden. Her son knew he did the only thing he could do, given all the circumstances, but he was far from content with the outcome.

I remember one patient with long-standing dementia. He spent each day at home under the watchful care of his wife. One day, she noticed that his face was drooping, and one arm and leg were not moving. Being familiar with the signs of stroke, she called 911 immediately, and the patient was brought to the ER. A CAT scan confirmed blockage of an artery in the brain, and our stroke team was called in. Now came the hard part. To treat the patient with clot-busting drugs was risky and expensive, but they might minimize the effects of the stroke. Not to treat him meant that the stroke would progress, but there was no way to tell how far, or whether it would be fatal. Eventually the decision was made to treat him. In the end, the patient was left partially paralyzed, although maybe not as badly as he might have been without treatment. But now he could no longer live at home. He was moved to a nursing home, where he died 10 months later of pneumonia. His wife still wonders whether she did the right thing. Would it have been better to bring him back home and let him die of the stroke? But would he have died? Would he have suffered even more? These are impossible questions. There is simply no way to know the right answers.

In the above examples, there was someone close to the patient who was able to make a decision. When there is no designated health care agent, situations can arise that challenge common sense. A dermatologist related the following story. He was called to a nursing home to see a 90-year-old woman with late-stage dementia who had developed a sore on her nose that wouldn't heal. He diagnosed basal cell cancer, a very slow-growing condition. His recommendation was to do nothing, given the patient's age and debility. More than likely the patient would die from other causes before the cancer would become dangerous. But because she didn't have an advance directive, medical decisions were made for her by the county's social services department. And because the social workers felt they had no right to do less than the maximum treatment available, the patient underwent several surgical procedures that were both expensive and uncomfortable. Given her condition, she had no understanding of what was being done to her. No one liked the situation, but no one could do anything to avoid it.

With the onset of dementia, a person must complete an advance directive straightaway while they are still competent to make their wishes known.

At the very least, given the prevalence of Alzheimer's disease, each of us ought to carefully consider what kind of care we'd want and under what circumstances. Advance directives are very helpful, but there are times when the forms simply cannot anticipate or account for every situation. MOLST/POLST forms can help too. Thus, although it may be difficult to do, talking candidly with our designated health care agent is essential. The answers won't be easy, but leaving these issues unaddressed will only make things worse for both the patient and the one who later has to make the decisions.

More and more, it's becoming clear that a serious discussion about care options is essential at the onset of dementia. There are numerous resources that offer guidance through the many aspects of diagnosing and managing of dementia. An excellent book is The 36-Hour Day.

At that point patients can still make their care wishes known and can imaginatively project into the future about what they might or might not want. It's hard enough to do this when the person still possesses most mental faculties, but waiting until they have become incompetent is worse. I know many couples who have outlined privately to each other what kind of care they'd want should dementia strike one of them. There are also cases of people who became aware of their dementia in its early phases and decided to commit suicide rather than face an inevitable decline.

Completing all the forms, having all the conversations, planning for every foreseeable eventuality can help. In the end, though, there are no easy answers or convenient ways to manage dementia, either on an individual or societal basis. But given the scale and severity of the problem, anything that can be of benefit ought to be done.

END-OF-LIFE CARE AND ECONOMICS

America's total medical costs hit a new record of $3.4 trillion [in 2016], according to the federal government. That's about 18 percent of the country's total GDP, meaning that one out of every six dollars we spent in 2016 went to health care. The national doctor bill dwarfs anything else we spend money on, including food, clothing, housing, or even our mighty military. For most people, the vast majority of all the health care they'll ever get comes near the hour of death. Hundreds of billions of dollars each year are spent treating Americans who are in the last weeks, or days, of life.
—T. R. REID, ATLANTIC, JUNE 15, 2017

There are more than 9,000 billing codes for individual procedures and units of care. But there is not a single billing code for patient adherence or improvement, or for helping patients stay well.
—CLAYTON M. CHRISTENSEN ET AL., THE INNOVATOR'S
PRESCRIPTION: A DISRUPTIVE SOLUTION FOR HEALTH CARE

There is no easy or comfortable way to talk about health care without talking about economics, and it's even harder to talk about those expenses in the context of end-of-life care.

In the United States, people get health insurance (for those who have it) either from a government program or from private insurance. Typically, private insurance is paid by employers, small and large, for whom this is an expensive and burdensome cost.

What's the basis for this? It goes back to World War II, when salaries couldn't be raised because of wartime wage and price controls. Instead, benefits were added. At that time, benefits didn't cost much, but now benefits account for a huge portion of a business's expenses, especially if that business also covers its retirees.

In our system, the closer you are to personally providing care to patients, the less money you make.

There is no longer any reason why this structure should remain. Americans should get jobs because they like them and have an opportunity to advance, not because a job provides good health insurance. Too many people stay in jobs they don't like only for the benefits. When a young adult gets a new job, we may not ask them if they like the work, their boss, or their coworkers, but we probably do ask them if health insurance came with it. This overriding concern stifles individual initiative and creativity and diverts companies from their primary mission.

Too many Americans are one serious illness away from financial ruin. Millions are still uninsured or underinsured. Health insurance companies, nonetheless, continue to reap huge profits, and their executives enjoy enormous salaries, bonuses, and stock options. Those who work on the front lines delivering the care, by contrast, are paid far less.

It's revealing that in the insurance world, the percentage of money spent on health care is termed a "loss ratio." In other words, insurers see the expenditures they make on our health as a loss, not as a benefit.

We've created a complex health care system whose economics are just about impossible for anyone to fully comprehend. It's a labyrinth of rules and regulations with money seemingly going in all directions except toward patient care. We spend more on health care than any other country in the world, yet our public health quality measures lag behind those of almost all other developed nations. We spend far more on sick care than on investing in prevention.

The good news is that most Americans are living longer and generally healthier lives. The technologies and advances that keep us going are increasingly expensive, and they are used more frequently. We seem to have, simultaneously, the best and worst of health care in the world.

How are health care costs managed? Typically, this is done through a variety of unpleasant means. The traditional ways to reduce health care costs are to limit access to care, shift more costs to the patient, and provide less service. Strict rules for what's allowed and what isn't are imposed by governments or insurance companies. Premiums paid by employers are raised, and payments to providers and health care delivery groups decrease. Patients pay more in copays and deductibles. These approaches are neither helpful nor supportive and typically lead to more red tape and confusion in our already overcomplicated and bureaucratic health care system.

IMPACT ON THE ECONOMY AND BUSINESSES

For most Americans today, 25% or more of all the health care dollars spent on their lives are spent in the last months of life. Money is spent keeping people alive far past any hope of their reasonable recovery, money that could be spent earlier, when the impact would be much greater in terms of quality and length of life. The number and proportion of those over age 65 in the United States is rising steadily. With the baby boom generation reaching old age, with its accompanying chronic diseases, health care costs will inevitably increase.

Some worry that advance directives for end-of-life planning are designed to save money. While it is likely that such planning will reduce health care costs for many people, in some cases that won't turn out to be true. Personally, I believe that a person's wishes must always come first and that economic impacts should be secondary. But there's no doubt that for many Americans who complete advance directives, care costs will decrease because of the choices most of us make. Most Americans would prefer to die at home or in hospice instead of in an intensive care unit once all life-sustaining treatments are exhausted. Remember that 80% of Americans die after a time of decline; only about 20% die suddenly. Every day not spent in a hospital or ICU saves $3,000 to $10,000.

Who pays for this care? Costs for end-of-life care may be paid by individuals, private insurance, Medicare, Medicaid, or other government programs.

About 85% of Americans who die are on some form of government health insurance, and of these Medicare is by far the largest single payer for end-of-life care. The annual Medicare budget is about $800 billion; spending in the last 6 months of life amounts to about 30% of this total, or $240 billion, and over 50% of that is spent in acute care hospitals. This means that of all the health care dollars spent throughout our lives, much of it is doled out for hospital care in the last months of life.

There are geographic variations to be considered as well. For example, Medicare spending for end of life in New York, New Jersey, and California averages 20% above the national average, while North Dakota, South Dakota, and Iowa are 25% below.

The "silver tsunami" of elderly persons in the United States will increase end-of-life care costs and consume more and more of the health care budget. The burden will be shifted to those who are working and contributing to Medicare via payroll taxes. Medicare, by itself, consumes about 15% of all federal spending today, and that's only going to increase.

We, as taxpayers, employers, and individuals, are all paying for this. Let's make sure we're paying for what we really want, and what most of us want is to die at home on our own terms. Advance directives not only provide a better dying experience for many, but they also reduce health care costs the right way: by empowering patients and respecting individual values.

According to Congressional Research Service (CRS) reports, the family members of loved ones "who died at a private home with hospice services were more likely to report a favorable dying experience." Of patients in a hospice program, more than 70% chose to die at home. But the CRS also noted that more of us are dying in the hospital (58%) or a nursing home (20%) than at home (22%). Expenses paid to institutions always cost more than expenditures for care at home. The questions for us to address are these: What portion of deaths in institutions would be more reasonably and less expensively managed at home, and how could that be achieved?

Medicaid, the federal/state program, is budgeted at about $600 billion a year, and the program is designed for those with limited means. About 75% of Medicaid funds go to 25% of Medicaid enrollees. Who belongs to this group? Mainly nursing home patients and the severely disabled. I'm not at all suggesting that we cut funding for them, but what I am suggesting is that these people often do not get the opportunity or support to complete advance directives and MOLST/POLST. If they did, they would likely want what most of us want: to take advantage of care when it's helpful and decline it when it isn't. The other 25% of Medicaid funds go to 75% of its enrollees. These are primarily children. Investing in children's health yields huge benefits over time and ultimately pays for itself several times over.

A few businesses are taking a look at how to promote advance directives with their employees. Some worry that their employees will see this as a cost-cutting measure, a reason to deny care when needed. That's understandable, given how much pressure there is already to limit access and choice. However, if done right, with sensitivity and forethought, it is a way to empower and support employees when they face serious illness themselves or in their families.

NATIONAL HEALTHCARE DECISIONS DAY

In 2014, Brent Pawlecki, MD (medical director for Goodyear Tire), and I wrote an article called "Companies Must Approach Advanced Health Events as a Business Issue" to acknowledge National Healthcare Decisions Day on April 16. What we wrote then still makes sense now:

> In the corporate world, every company has a chief financial officer charged with ensuring that the organization meets all tax and accounting mandates and to report the data to officers of the company, shareholders, employees and the general public. Yet, while organizations expend great effort addressing these matters, many miss another opportunity to protect their employees' well-being by failing to talk about end-of-life care. Most companies consider advanced illness to be a private matter. But in fact, this hands-off approach most assuredly affects the financial health of any organization—and the emotional well-being of its workforce.
>
> Beyond its direct impact on individuals' health and well-being, advanced illness can take a heavy economic toll, including its effects on productivity, health and benefits costs, employee potential and engagement. According to the MetLife Mature Market Institute study, the total estimated cost to employers for all full-time employed caregivers is a staggering $33.6 billion. The average cost per employee for caregiving responsibilities ranges from $2,100 to $2,400.
>
> The challenges of dealing with a loved one's advanced illness also affects worker productivity. While almost all companies claim that their most valuable assets are their employees, most businesses have not yet fully recognized the impact of advanced illness on their employees' performance. Family caregivers provide more than 80 percent of long-term care services in the United States (i.e., services for advanced illness), and more than

73 percent of those caregivers are employed while caring for a family member. As the population ages ("the silver tsunami"), this number will only continue to increase.

Further data indicates that the percentage of adults with the dual role of caregiver/employee rose from 62 percent in 2005 to 69 percent in 2009. These employees sometimes arrived late to work, left early, or took time off during the day to provide care. A survey by one Fortune 500 corporation of its caregiving employees revealed that one in five were actively considering leaving the workplace because of their caregiving duties— a potential huge loss of talent.

In response to both the economic and emotional costs of dealing with advanced illness, some employers—such as GE, Goodyear, IBM, PepsiCo, and Pitney Bowes—have begun to address advanced illness as part of the normal course of life event planning along with help organizing college funds or retirement plans. These employers incorporate the appropriate tools as part of their health and wellness offerings, and according to many employee surveys, their employees appreciate this recognition of reality. . . .

Every year, April 16 marks National Healthcare Decisions Day, appropriately corresponding to the deadlines of tax season. This event provides a perfect opportunity for individuals and companies to begin the discussion about this challenging but important issue. To some individuals, the thought of planning for a death may seem a bit macabre. In fact, it's not planning that too often makes the macabre a reality for individuals and for their loved ones.

Employers cannot erase the tremendous challenges that employees face as caregivers or during a health crisis. However, they can foster a positive and empowering environment that supports employees with the plans and tools that will help ease this burden. . . . On National Healthcare Decisions Day, businesses should take the lead. It's the right and responsible thing to do, entirely consistent with sound management policies, good for the well-being of their employees, and best for the bottom line.

DOING IT RIGHT: LA CROSSE, WISCONSIN

Can these changes in culture and habits actually happen? To answer that, it's worth taking a look at the situation in La Crosse, Wisconsin.

La Crosse is the city center of a metropolitan area of about 140,000 people. Starting in the 1990s, concerned citizens who had recently dealt with family deaths joined with a few dedicated health care professionals to begin promoting discussions about end-of-life care. This led to an effort by the medical, legal, business, and faith communities to encourage the completion of advance directives. This campaign was supported by the Gundersen Health System, the dominant health care system in the area. Over time, the rate of completion of advance directives rose. Now over 96% of the La Crosse adult population has completed these forms. A community resource called Respecting Choices (respecting choices.org) helps empower citizens for a broad range of health care decisions.

Talking about death is not a taboo subject there. It is the norm. It's just one of the things that everyone does from time to time as part of the responsibility of being a citizen in a community. The results are clear. According to the Dartmouth Atlas of Health Care, La Crosse spends about 30% to 40% less on end-of-life care than any other place in the United States. More importantly, La Crosse residents are managing their dying experience according to their own wishes. Family stress and guilt are reduced. If there is such a thing as a good end-of-life care template, the people in La Crosse have achieved it. The question for the rest of us should be, Why aren't we making this happen everywhere?

8

Assisted Suicide, Assisted Dying, and VSED

Numbing the pain for a while will make it worse when you finally feel it.
—J. K. ROWLING, HARRY POTTER AND THE GOBLET OF FIRE

Turn your wounds into wisdom.
—OPRAH WINFREY

What is the right course to take when pain is intractable and there is no hope for recovery? Two scenarios that are emotionally charged and extensively covered by the media are assisted suicide and assisted dying. There's a critical difference between assisted suicide and assisted dying. In assisted suicide, a person no longer wants to live. In assisted dying, a person wishes they could.

ASSISTED SUICIDE

Assisted suicide is when one person helps another person end their own life. The assistance can be administering a lethal dose of medicine or killing someone by another method. The notoriety of Dr. Jack Kevorkian brought this issue to public attention in a sensational way. Assisted suicide in the form of euthanasia or "mercy killing" is not legal in the United States. This is not to be confused with assisted dying, described in the next section, which is allowed in some states.

There are ways that individuals can direct their care without resorting to problematic measures that raise complex ethical and legal issues. The best, easiest, and legal way that covers most situations is to complete an advance directive.

It is important to point out that assisted suicide does not include the case of someone who chooses to forgo treatment and dies a natural death when there is no expectation of recovery.

ASSISTED DYING

> Mental pain is less dramatic than physical pain, but it is more common and also more hard to bear. The frequent attempt to conceal mental pain increases the burden: it is easier to say "My tooth is aching" than to say "My heart is broken."
> —C. S. LEWIS, THE PROBLEM OF PAIN

The human body can be both fragile and resilient at the same time, and there are significant individual variations based on factors we don't understand. For example, people who smoke have a much higher incidence of cancer and lung problems, but there are some who smoke for decades and don't seem to be damaged. It's the same with alcohol abuse. Most suffer the ravages of excessive drinking, but there are a few who don't. Obviously, genetics and other circumstances play a role. Some people get an illness and go fast. There are others who, despite severe illness, linger for decades.

Today, several countries and seven US states (California, Colorado, Hawaii, Montana, Oregon, Vermont, and Washington) and the District of Columbia allow terminally ill patients to take their own life. Similar legislation is being considered in several other states. While this is a highly controversial topic, a 2018 Gallup poll showed that 72% of Americans across all demographic groups favor the availability of some sort of assisted dying process. Nearly 60% of physicians believe that this should be legal as well.

Other nations including Canada, the Netherlands, Japan, Australia, Colombia, South Korea, Switzerland, Uruguay, and Belgium have adopted death-with-dignity laws.

These laws vary from country to country, consistent with national values and culture. For example, Belgium has one of the most permissive laws, allowing euthanasia as well as assisted suicide even for non-terminal conditions. In contrast, Uruguay maintains the illegality of assisted suicide but authorizes judges to "forgo punishment of a person whose previous life has been honorable where he commits a homicide motivated by compassion, induced by repeated requests of the victim."

The human body is both fragile and resilient at the same time.

In the United States, the legislation that allows for assisted dying varies by state but has some common features. To qualify for the right, a person has to be a resident of the state and have a terminal condition. There is a defined process by which the person makes the request and by which a physician—or more than one physician—documents the patient's condition. There is a waiting period between the time of the request and the time of authorization. The physician is then allowed to write a prescription for the lethal medications. These typically include a sedative, an anti-nausea medicine, and other medicines that work in different ways to slow down and eventually stop breathing or stop the heart from beating. Only the patient can administer the medicine; it cannot be given to them by another person. When properly done, the patient will die within a few minutes or a few hours.

ASSISTED DYING: PROS AND CONS

Assisted dying is a hot topic, and discussing it gets our juices flowing. It's much better cocktail party conversation to argue about the pros and cons of assisted dying than to chat about completing boring paperwork, like advance directives. Just like it's more stimulating to discuss the pros and cons of the death penalty, with various hypotheticals, than to engage in an exploration of why violent crime occurs and how to prevent it.

Here are some of the pro and con arguments about assisted dying:

Pro:

— It's a personal decision as are other key decisions in life, and these are best left to the individual involved.

— Death with dignity is a human right.

— Physicians are not directly involved in the administration of the drugs, so this does not violate any professional ethics.

— The laws that allow it provide sufficient process and protection.

— There is no evidence that passing these laws has led to any abuses in the states that have, nor is there any evidence of this from the other countries where assisted dying is allowed.

— Despite best efforts and a full range of resources, there are patients (such as Brittany Maynard, whose story follows) for whom this is the only reasonable course of action.

Con:

— Authorizing dying will promote more suicides.

— Life is sacred and must be honored.

— There are many ways that end-of-life care and the management of critical illness can be done so that assisted dying is not needed.

— Engaging in this activity by any health professional, directly or indirectly, runs counter to the credo "do no harm."

— These laws lead us down a slippery slope where euthanasia becomes acceptable for people who are deemed less desirable by society.

— No matter how tight the legislation, there will always be a financial interest at stake, whether for families or insurance companies.

It's not being dead that frightens most of us. After all, every human being before us has managed to die, and all of us will too someday. It's the process of getting there.

BRITTANY MAYNARD TELLS HER STORY

No amount of planning is foolproof or will accommodate every circumstance. There are always going to be outliers who don't fit into any convenient paradigm or medical care plan. Brittany Maynard was just such a case.

Brittany was a 29-year-old woman from California, tragically afflicted with terminal brain cancer. She moved to Oregon to take advantage of the state's death-with-dignity law, and she ended her life there. There is no better way to understand her decision-making process than to read her own words:

On New Year's Day, after months of suffering from debilitating headaches, I learned that I had brain cancer. I was 29 years old. I'd been married for just over a year. My husband and I were trying for a family. Our lives devolved into hospital stays, doctor consultations and medical research. Nine days after my initial diagnoses, I had a partial craniotomy and a partial resection of my temporal lobe. Both surgeries were an effort to stop the growth of my tumor.

In April, I learned that not only had my tumor come back, but it was more aggressive. Doctors gave me a prognosis of six months to live.

Because my tumor is so large, doctors prescribed full brain radiation. I read about the side effects: The hair on my scalp would have been singed off. My scalp would be left covered with first-degree burns. My quality of life, as I knew it, would be gone.

After months of research, my family and I reached a heart-breaking conclusion: There is no treatment that would save my life, and the recommended treatments would have destroyed the time I had left.

I considered passing away in hospice care at my San Francisco Bay–area home. But even with palliative medication, I could develop potentially morphine-resistant pain and suffer personality changes and verbal, cognitive, and motor loss of virtually any kind.

Because the rest of my body is young and healthy, I am likely to physically hang on for a long time even though cancer is eating my mind. I probably would have suffered in hospice care for weeks or even months. And my family would have had to watch that.

I did not want this nightmare scenario for my family, so I started researching death with dignity. It is an end-of-life option

for mentally competent, terminally ill patients with a prognosis of six months or less to live. It would enable me to use the
medical practice of aid in dying: I could request and receive a
prescription from a physician for medication that I could self-
ingest to end my dying process if it becomes unbearable.

I quickly decided that death with dignity was the best option
for me and my family. We had to uproot from California to
Oregon, because Oregon is one of only five states where death
with dignity is authorized. I met the criteria for death with dignity in Oregon, but establishing residency in the state to make
use of the law required a monumental number of changes. I had
to find new physicians, establish residency in Portland, search
for a new home, obtain a new driver's license, change my voter
registration and enlist people to take care of our animals, and my
husband, Dan, had to take a leave of absence from his job. The
vast majority of families do not have the flexibility, resources,
and time to make all these changes.

I've had the medication for weeks. I am not suicidal. If I
were, I would have consumed that medication long ago. I do not
want to die. But I am dying. And I want to die on my own terms.

I would not tell anyone else that he or she should choose
death with dignity. My question is: Who has the right to tell
me that I don't deserve this choice? That I deserve to suffer
for weeks or months in tremendous amounts of physical and
emotional pain? Why should anyone have the right to make that
choice for me?

Now that I've had the prescription filled and it's in my possession, I have experienced a tremendous sense of relief. And if
I decide to change my mind about taking the medication, I will
not take it.

Having this choice at the end of my life has become incredibly important. It has given me a sense of peace during a
tumultuous time that otherwise would be dominated by fear,
uncertainty and pain.

Now, I'm able to move forward in my remaining days or weeks I have on this beautiful Earth, to seek joy and love and to spend time traveling to outdoor wonders of nature with those I love. And I know that I have a safety net.

I plan to celebrate my husband's birthday on October 26 with him and our family. Unless my condition improves dramatically, I will look to pass soon thereafter. I hope for the sake of my fellow American citizens that I'll never meet that this option is available to you. If you ever find yourself walking a mile in my shoes, I hope that you would at least be given the same choice and that no one tries to take it from you.

When my suffering becomes too great, I can say to all those I love, "I love you; come be by my side, and come say goodbye as I pass into whatever's next." I will die upstairs in my bedroom with my husband, mother, stepfather and best friend by my side and pass peacefully. I can't imagine trying to rob anyone else of that choice.

THE LEGISLATION

I've sat in legislative hearings on these bills in Maryland. The hearings went on for hours, and everyone who spoke—on all sides—was sincere and compelling. I listened carefully to everyone and reviewed the legislative language in detail. Although the bills never came up for a vote during my time in the legislature, here's my position on this.

I believe that many of the concerns raised on all sides can be solved by doing things right now that are legal and uncontroversial. The problem is that most of us don't follow the basic steps: complete advance directives, use palliative care and hospice early, plan for final days, treat pain effectively, work with providers to complete MOLST/POLST forms, and manage anxiety and depression. Sadly, we fall short in all these areas. If these were part of our routines as responsible adults and clinicians, my guess is that 99% of the issues that worry all of us would be resolved.

I'd want to be sure that any proposed assisted dying bill would require a person to have gone through a number of steps first. These would include completing an advance directive, evaluation by a palliative care specialist, and evaluation by hospice. Pain should be reduced to the greatest extent possible, and all measures for comfort would be used. If needed, any mental health condition, such as depression, should be treated. I'd also want to make sure that there were sufficient and multiple time lags between the various steps so that someone would not act on any impulsive decision.

All the legislation enacted in the United States so far meets these standards. In Oregon, for example, about 65% (148 out of 249) of the people who went through the process to get a prescription for lethal medication actually took it. Here are other statistics from the Oregon experience about the citizens who participated in the program: 79.2% were over the age of 65, with the median age being 74; 62.5% had cancer; 90.5% were in hospice care at the time of death; 88.6% died at home; and 99.3% had some form of insurance. These numbers have been consistent since the establishment of the program.

In my 24 years in the Maryland legislature, I heard arguments against many issues where the bill in question eventually passed, and then none of the predicted dire consequences came true.

This was brought home to me in my first legislative session in 1995. There was an issue for which every member was lobbied intensively every day. For the bill in question, we were told that if we voted for it, its passage would be a major step forward for public health, that it would save lives and reduce health care costs. Those in opposition said that the bill would seriously damage several key economic sectors in Maryland, especially the hospitality industry (restaurants, hotels, tourism); jobs would be lost, and the tax base eroded. Furthermore, the legislation was a governmental overstep into personal rights that would dictate right and wrong behaviors in a free society.

_____

The slippery slope never materialized for smoking bans. Why would passing a carefully written bill for assisted dying be different?

_____

What was this bill? It was to ban smoking in restaurants. Eventually we passed the bill, and none of the dire predictions came to pass. In fact, the opposite occurred. More people went out to eat, and business flourished. Nonetheless, it took more than 10 years to ban smoking in bars as well, and the arguments against it were pretty much the same, as was the outcome.

In all these cases and many others, the slippery slope never materialized.

That's why, in the end, I would have voted for a carefully written assisted dying bill, one providing options at the end of life that would be beneficial for the relatively few people whose circumstances couldn't be managed in any other way.

VSED

Another choice is known as VSED, which stands for "voluntarily stopping eating and drinking." While many would never consider it, some choose to use this method to hasten death.

John Rehm, the husband of Diane Rehm, a radio host on National Public Radio, was suffering from Parkinson's disease. He had asked his physician for medication to help him die, but John's request was denied, as it was illegal. So he stopped ingesting water and nutrition. Diane Rehm shares her perspective on her husband's decision in her book *When My Time Comes*.

If you've ever fasted, you know how difficult it can be. But when people are near death, their need for food and water diminishes, and refusing them seems to be much easier. Studies from the Netherlands indicated that the median time for death to occur was 7 days and that for most patients the process unfolded as they had wanted.

When 94-year-old Rosemary Bowen told her family that she had decided on VSED, they tried to dissuade her. But when it became clear that Rosemary was determined to proceed, her daughter Mary Beth Bowen documented her mother's experience in a short film, *Leaving Life on My Own Terms*. It is a moving record of her mother's reasoning, determination, and equanimity. Rosemary Bowen would have preferred to take medication, but since that was not a legal option, she chose VSED.

> It has been said, "time heals all wounds." I do not agree. The wounds remain. In time, the mind, protecting its sanity, covers them with scar tissue and the pain lessens. But it is never gone.
> —ROSE FITZGERALD KENNEDY

> There is a saying in Tibetan, "Tragedy should be utilized as a source of strength." No matter what sort of difficulties, how painful experience is, if we lose our hope, that's our real disaster.
> —DALAI LAMA XIV

9

Pain, Anxiety, and
Drugs, Drugs, Drugs

———

I have absolutely no pleasure in the stimulants in which I some-times so madly indulge. It has not been in the pursuit of pleasure that I have periled life and reputation and reason. It has been the desperate attempt to escape from torturing memories, from a sense of insupportable loneliness and a dread of some strange impending doom.

—Edgar Allan Poe

THE START OF THE "WAR ON DRUGS"

Fear of pain is a major concern when people are facing end-of-life choices. In fact, this fear drives much of the activism around the assisted dying issue. The truth is that there are many methods to alleviate pain and anxiety, but some of these are controversial.

Today we live in the midst of an opioid crisis, especially in the United States. More Americans died from drug overdoses in 2017 than died in the entire Vietnam War, and over the past few years more have died annually from drug overdoses than from AIDS, gun deaths, and car deaths combined. It's worth reviewing some of the history of how this came about.

The modern "War on Drugs" began in 1970 with the administration of President Richard Nixon. His director of domestic policy, John Ehrlichman, revealed in a 1994 interview published in *Harper's* magazine what the thinking really was:

> *Fear of pain drives much of the activism around the assisted dying issue.*

> You want to know what this was really all about? The Nixon campaign in 1968, and the Nixon White House after that, had two enemies: the antiwar left and black people. You understand what I'm saying? We knew we couldn't make it illegal to be either against the war or black, but by getting the public to associate the hippies with marijuana and blacks with heroin, and then criminalizing both heavily, we could disrupt those communities. We could arrest their leaders, raid their homes, break up their meetings, and vilify them night after night on the evening news. Did we know we were lying about the drugs? Of course we did.

Sadly, that political policy worked. Many people were imprisoned for possession of small amounts of drugs, and societal and cultural divisions were created that exist to this day.

AN ER DOCTOR–LEGISLATOR'S APPROACH

From my perspective as a clinician and as a legislator, the War on Drugs is an epic policy failure. After 50 years into the war, there is not one single measurable outcome that shows improvement. In fact, everything is worse. Despite all the money spent and all the lives lost and the millions imprisoned, there are more drug users, more overdose deaths, more deadly diseases spread such as HIV and hepatitis, more violence at home and overseas, pervasive corruption, vast money laundering schemes, more families and communities torn apart, and escalating costs for taxpayers.

I'm sure that many people were well intentioned in their fight against substance abuse, but the policies focused much more on law enforcement than on treatment. None of these efforts has decreased drug abuse, and there's not a shred of evidence that continuing to do the same thing will lead to a different outcome. Worse yet, proven public health measures—such as sites for opioid overdose and infectious disease prevention—have yet to become legal in the United States.

There has finally been some recognition that more access to treatment is needed, but that's been slow in coming. The first bill I sponsored to promote substance abuse treatment was in 1998. People ask me why I thought to introduce a bill so many years ago, before the rest of the country came to acknowledge that there was a crisis. The answer is easy: I just noted what was happening to patients who came to the emergency room for care. More and more visits were related to drug use. This legislation was enacted, and it made some progress, but it was far from enough.

Here's how being an ER doctor gave me a perspective not readily available to others. When finishing the documentation and medical notes on a patient's chart, I enter the final diagnosis on the medical record. Typically, this reflects the somatic problem, not the underlying reason for the visit. For example, I might treat an intravenous substance abuser for a skin abscess (pus pocket infection under the skin) caused by using a dirty needle. Treating it might be a straightforward procedure, or it might be a complicated one. But the final diagnosis—the one used for billing and data collection—would be "abscess." The diagnosis would be the same for someone who had scraped a knee that later became infected.

One of the ways I prepared for the legislative bill hearing in 1998 was to study the ER charts of patients who came in with no insurance. Some clinically savvy colleagues and I read the complete charts of this group. We found that 60% to 70% of the patients had come there for drug use, but that term didn't show up in the final diagnoses. We found evidence for this because we knew how to read doctors' and nurses' medical notes. We might find the abbreviation "IVDA" (intravenous drug abuse) recorded, or the result of a toxicology screen would be positive for opiates; the physical exam might note "needle tracks" (scars on the forearms from repeated drug injection), or the history would record "drug use." That information helped convince my legislative colleagues that addiction treatment would reduce uncompensated care in the ER, which could be a step toward lowering the fiscal burden for taxpayers and insurance buyers.

Understanding this social and political backdrop helps explain our current circumstances.

> I don't like to overdose. Call me old-fashioned.
> —CHELSEA HANDLER

> Drugs are a bet with your mind.
> —JIM MORRISON

TREATING PAIN AND ANXIETY

No one wants to suffer needlessly, and modern medicines and pain management techniques have made tremendous progress in relieving discomfort. There are a variety of medicines used to treat people with serious and advanced illness. Sometimes these medicines are given to help patients endure difficult treatments or side effects. Sometimes they are used to relieve the pain that comes in dying. Patients and their families may be anxious about taking these medicines because they fear dependency, side effects, and over-sedation. These concerns are legitimate, but all can be addressed.

NONPHARMACOLOGIC METHODS
AND OTC MEDICATIONS

There are methods of treating pain that do not involve medication. These include ice or heat, rest, weight reduction, physical therapy, acupuncture, massage, wraps, splints, crutches, prayer, meditation, exercise, music, spending time outdoors in nature, and self-hypnosis. These should be considered equally with pharmacology as treatment options. I believe that all these modalities can be used. They are often complementary and work together well in ways we may not fully understand. All patients should have the opportunity to find what works best for them individually.

Among over-the-counter, or OTC, medicines for treating pain, the options are straightforward. To start with, there's aspirin, an excellent pain medicine with some side effects, most notably upset stomach. Then there's acetaminophen (Tylenol), also an effective pain medicine.

The next group is nonsteroidal anti-inflammatory drugs (NSAIDs), such as ibuprofen (Motrin) and naproxen (Aleve). Both aspirin and NSAIDs relieve pain, reduce inflammation, and lower fevers. Acetaminophen relieves pain and lowers fevers but does not reduce inflammation. On a biochemical level, aspirin and the NSAIDs work similarly and have the same side effects, but acetaminophen works on a different biochemical pathway. That's why I often recommend to patients with pain problems that they try both ibuprofen (or aspirin) and acetaminophen in the following regimen. I suggest they take one of each to start; then take one 4 hours later and the other 4 hours after that, and so on. That way they are getting pain relief by both mechanisms but reduce the risks of side effects since they are taking only half the full dose. This is the drug regimen I use personally, and it's the one I recommend to my friends and family for standard aches and pains and minor injuries.

Aspirin, NSAIDs, and acetaminophen are all available without a prescription from your local drugstore or supermarket. Nonetheless, these medicines all have side effects and risks, especially if too many are taken, and they can interact adversely with other medicines, alcohol, and drugs.

NARCOTICS, OPIOIDS, SEDATIVES, AND TRANQUILIZERS

There may be some confusion between the terms "opioid" and "narcotic." The terms are generally used interchangeably now, but there is a technical difference. Opioids are medicines developed from or based on opium derived from the opium poppy. Many opioids today are made synthetically. They relieve pain and lead to sleep. The term "narcotic" refers to medicines that encourage sleep (narcosis). For example, diazepam (Valium) has narcotic properties, but it is not an opioid. In other words, all opioids have narcotic properties, but not all narcotics are opioids.

All the opioid medicines are variants of one another, and in the final analysis, they work through our body's opioid receptor system. These receptors are present in various cells throughout the body, and they are activated when an opioid drug connects with them. This starts a chemical and electrical cascade that leads to pain relief. Knowing that external substances had this effect led to the insight that there must be internal ones as well. Our bodies' internal opioid system is regulated by endorphins, opioid-like compounds that we make for ourselves.

Opioids, as everyone should be aware, have numerous risks, ranging from the inconvenient to the potentially deadly. Humans have a long and complicated history with them. The more commonly known ones are heroin, morphine, fentanyl, hydromorphone (Dilaudid), codeine, hydrocodone (often combined with acetaminophen in medicines like Vicodin and Norco), and Oxy-Contin (extended-release oxycodone). Drugs in this class are sometimes abused, especially heroin, which provides a "rush" in addition to pain relief.

Opioids relieve pain effectively, especially acute pain or cancer pain, but people who take them run the risk of developing an addiction. However, when pharmaceutically approved drugs are used carefully for pain management, these medicines don't have to be addictive. Once pain is controlled, the doses should be reduced. There are side effects, as happens with almost any medicine, and the most common ones with opioids (sometimes called opiates) are constipation and sleepiness. But, again, with careful dosage and by avoiding long-term use, these side effects can be minimized.

Furthermore, research demonstrates a difference in how medical practitioners treat people of different backgrounds when it comes to pain. Minorities are less likely to receive adequate pain relief compared with whites, and women are less likely to get pain medicines than men. Whether this bias is intentional or not, the impact is real, and practitioners and health organizations are engaged in strategies to see that everyone gets the proper level of care.

Opioids can be given by mouth, skin patch, suppository, or by injection. Individuals may have a preferred method of administration. These medicines can be safely given at home, hospital, nursing home, or hospice. Regardless of the route of administration, these drugs work the same way via the human body's built-in opiate receptors.

I had one patient who was almost constantly in moderate to severe pain from advanced disease, and he resisted the use of opioids. He was depressed and had trouble performing at his part-time job. He finally gave in, however, and was started on morphine. Almost immediately, his pain was relieved, and he began to sleep better. His mood lightened, and his thinking improved. He functioned better in every aspect of life and later told me that he wished he'd started a pain relief program sooner. Once his pain was controlled, he was weaned off opioids and did well.

Morphine also helps relieve the symptoms of shortness of breath, sometimes referred to as "air hunger." This seems paradoxical in that too much morphine slows or stops breathing. Yet it works for many patients, as it did for Michael Martinez (chapter 2).

An acceptance of coming death may diminish some people's resistance to using opioids for pain relief. After all, what are the risks when a patient is at the end of life? Is there a need to worry about addiction when someone has only a few months to live?

It's not the drug that is good or bad; it's the context of its use.

Sedatives and tranquilizers (such as diazepam) are another class of medications that may be used. These medications can help with anxiety, sleep, and mood disorders, all common symptoms in those with a serious illness. Again, when used responsibly, the benefits outweigh the risks. Taking narcotics, opioids, and sedatives at the same time, or with alcohol, can be dangerous and should be avoided.

Hopefully, patients with an advanced illness are cared for by a team of professionals including doctors, nurses, and pharmacists. When that is the case, most pain and anxiety can be safely managed.

A fine line separates symptom relief, however, from speeding the death process. When does effective pain relief become assisted dying, which is a crime in some states? The state has an interest in protecting its citizens' lives, but laws can have a chilling effect on caregivers. A doctor perceived to be "over-prescribing" opioids for pain, even at the request of a patient, could face criminal or civil charges.

For me, it's not the drug; it's the context of its use. Any drug is a substance without any moral standing of its own. Picture a bottle with 25 opioid pills. Is that good or bad? If this bottle belongs to a person with severe bone pain from metastatic cancer, then the drug is entirely appropriate. But if the bottle is stolen and its contents sold on the street for cash, the situation is entirely different. We cannot say that opioids are either "bad" or "good" in all possible situations. Instead, these medicines ought to be seen as tools, useful in some situations but posing significant risks.

THE PAIN ISSUE

In the late 1990s and early 2000s, the pain issue came to the forefront of public discussion and the media. The battle cry was that patients were not getting enough relief for their pain and that providers were ignoring this problem. In my experience, health care providers—nurses, physicians, dentists, pharmacists, physician assistants, paramedics—were not ignoring their patients' pain or being insensitive to their suffering. Since then, we've learned that much of this ballyhoo was created and fueled by drug companies, notably Purdue Pharmaceuticals, that wanted to sell more OxyContin. Purdue is now being sued by states on behalf of their citizens for its deceitful role in creating the current opioid addiction crisis, and Purdue has been forced to pay billions in settlements.

I saw this directly as a legislator. Bills were introduced in Maryland and in many other states to declare pain the "fifth vital sign" alongside the classic four vital signs: pulse, blood pressure, temperature, and respiratory rate. I opposed all of these bills because I saw them as an unnecessary intrusion on medical practice, and I had firsthand experience to know that pain was being recognized and treated responsibly. But at the time I didn't know about the corporate forces pushing this agenda forward.

I'm not always prescient, but I knew that this whole effort was wrong. I spoke out against the "pain bills," trying to avoid coming off as a heartless doctor who didn't care about patient suffering. I tried to tone down the response in my hospital, but the pressure from outside forces was relentless.

Fortunately in Maryland almost all these bills were defeated. But a new attitude toward pain relief was created that permeated clinical decision-making for years to come.

The Joint Commission on Accreditation of Healthcare Organizations (JCAHO) got on-board with the "pain issue." JCAHO accreditation is essential for hospitals that expect to get paid by Medicare and other payers, so this issue became important. Nurses were instructed to ask patients regularly about their pain, often having them rate it on a scale of 1 to 10 or having them point to one in a series of cartoon faces, from smiling to grimacing, to indicate their level of discomfort. Nurses would then call and ask doctors to prescribe pain meds for their patients.

Likewise, doctors were evaluated for how they treated pain. We were all pressured to ask patients frequently about pain, and the medical team responded promptly by medicating them. This was a subject at department meetings and hospital-wide conferences. Medical seminars were devoted to this, and pain evaluation and treatment became a hot topic.

Hospital surveys of patients started to include pain scores. If the scores were too low, then corrective steps were taken. Sometimes that meant a one-on-one discussion with your supervisor as "motivation" for bringing your scores up to an acceptable level.

Licensing boards got involved too. It's critical to note that licensing boards have tremendous influence because they have the power to limit or terminate someone's license to practice medicine, effectively ending their career.

In Maryland, the newsletter from the licensing board for physicians began to include articles about pain and the need to treat it. The board even provided a hotline number and contact information for speakers who'd come to your hospital to talk about pain and the need for medication. Only later was it recognized that the hotline connected callers to a Purdue Pharmaceuticals representative and that the speakers were physicians paid by Purdue. I eventually used those Maryland Board of Medicine newsletters in arguing for legislation to limit the board to its appropriate tasks, and that bill was enacted.

I remember one of those Purdue-sponsored conferences. We were told that OxyContin was not addictive. It was implied that the pain—by some miraculous method—sort of soaked up the medication, so the drug would disappear and no one would get addicted. It's hard to write this now without feeling disgusted because so much harm was done. All this wasn't by accident. It was part of an organized plan to sell as much product as possible. The strategy worked. Opioid prescriptions increased, and the country became awash in dangerous, addictive drugs.

The consequences of this terrible approach rippled through society. When people couldn't continue to get prescribed opioids, some hit the street to buy illicit heroin, fentanyl, or whatever they could get to maintain their habit.

When I evaluate patients with pain, I have to assess several things at the same time. My decision isn't hard when the injury (such as a broken arm) or illness (a kidney stone or a heart attack) is obvious. It can be equally obvious, at times, when a patient is much more dramatic about their pain than is consistent with their physical condition. There are people who try to manipulate prescribers (sometimes with success, sometimes not) into writing prescriptions for opioids.

Sometimes the cases are more difficult to evaluate. What about a person who is complaining of an episode of worsening chronic back pain? They are suffering and look miserable. They will have often gone through most other options. Adding opioids may provide some short-term relief, but for an ongoing condition, the risks with continued opioid use multiply.

My personal experience taking opioids is limited. Once I had a broken tooth, and it was incredibly painful. I loaded up on acetaminophen and ibuprofen, but that didn't work. It was a Friday night, and I knew I couldn't see a dentist until Monday. At least my dentist was on-call and available, so I explained the situation.

I couldn't rest or sleep or do anything, and he gave me a prescription for 10 pills of short-acting oxycodone. It worked, and on Monday he saw me in his office. I had taken only a few of the pills, but it made all the difference. I was careful too. I didn't mix them with any other medicines and didn't drive when under their influence. I did get a little constipated, a common side effect, so I walked and drank lots of water to help minimize that.

There are some new medication options, but these are tricky to use and require close monitoring. The most notable ones are gabapentin (Neurontin), pregabalin (Lyrica), and duloxetine (Cymbalta). These medicines are used for neuropathic pain, like that from diabetes or shingles or fibromyalgia. Some doctors feel they are over-marketed and overused and not very effective.

On the issue of pain, the pendulum has swung back and forth. First, we were told that there was too much untreated pain and that clinicians needed to prescribe more drugs. And so they did. Today the message is that it's time to rein in opioid and narcotic prescribing, and a host of measures have been put in place. For example, each state now has a prescription drug monitoring program that monitors every scheduled drug prescription. (A "scheduled" drug is a controlled substance; more on that below.) Unfortunately, this has created another problem. There are patients who truly need pain- and anxiety-relieving medications who are not getting them, particularly those at the end of life. Hopefully, we'll be able to find the proper balance of using these important medications.

Moreover, too many people with an addiction disorder can't get treatment when they need it. For almost all the medical conditions for which people come to an ER, I have many resources to rely on as appropriate. I can treat the patient, admit them to the hospital, call in a specialist for consultation, or direct them to outpatient services. But all too often, when a patient presents with a substance abuse disorder and is motivated to seek treatment, the best I can offer is a sheet of paper with a list of treatment centers. I have to hope that the patient will still be motivated the next morning to make the call and that the center will have an opening for them. Persons with substance abuse disorders, however, tend to be focused on their next fix, not on planning for a medical appointment sometime in the future. For these patients, it's important to act while they are motivated to get treatment. I ought to be able to get them into proper care right then, as I would for any other patient condition. But that's not possible. Not surprisingly, too few of these patients get the treatment they need.

As access to prescription opioids has tightened, illegal sources are the only ones left. That drives a huge amount of crime in our country. By some estimates, more than 80% of all crime is related to drugs.

THE HOW AND WHY OF THE US ADDICTION EPIDEMIC

I used to have a drug problem, now I make enough money.
—DAVID LEE ROTH

We are confronting a global drug market, with product grown overseas and shipped into the United States on an industrial scale, with a distribution system that reaches every community. The billions in cash from sales is laundered through banks and then sent back overseas to drug cartels often run by terrorist organizations. The net result is this: we are sticking to a policy that is destroying our citizenry from the inside while financing our enemies who would destroy us from the outside.

There is a deeper question that we've collectively been reluctant to ask: Why are so many Americans turning to drugs for escape? Joaquín "El Chapo" Guzmán had an interesting perspective on this. When asked why he sold drugs, he responded, "If there was no consumption, there would be no sales." In other words, El Chapo saw himself as a businessman supplying a product we wanted. Why do we want this product? What is the void in our culture that leads people across all demographics to turn to drugs?

Here's my theory. Our culture celebrates values that are ultimately not satisfying. These include our obsession with money, acquiring objects, physical appearance, and status. Maybe that's why some people who by those standards are incredibly successful nonetheless suffer from drug use, depression, marital problems, and suicidal tendencies.

There's a classic scientific experiment that you may have heard about. In it, a rat was put in a cage with two levers. One dispensed drugs, the other food. Rat after rat put in the cage with the same choice kept pushing the drug lever until it either overdosed or starved to death. The conclusion we were to draw is that drugs are bad and automatically addictive. But that experiment was redone with a twist by Dr. Bruce Alexander. He created a "rat park," a setting that had everything rats like: food, toys, tunnels, and other rats. In that setting, few rats pushed the drug lever. What we can conclude from that result is that the availability of drugs is not what leads to addiction. Rather, it's the lack of connection. The opposite of addiction is not just sobriety; it's community. I've talked with thousands of persons with substance abuse disorders, and I've asked them about their childhood and their life situation. This is often in the context of an ER visit, but it's more like chatting than a formal interview. Almost all of these people have had some terrible things happen to them. Many were victims of childhood beatings or sexual abuse, were not encouraged to learn in school, often went to bed hungry, and witnessed domestic violence. There were some for whom I thought, "If that were my life, I might be using drugs too. Anything to escape."

In addition to all the other measures being recommended to address the addiction epidemic, our society needs to take a hard look at itself. Perhaps other values need to be encouraged such as

> *The opposite of addiction is not just sobriety; it's community.*

helping neighbors, demonstrating compassion, finding meaningful (not just profitable) work, tolerating differences, having civil discourse, and engaging with our communities. These are not just nice ideas; they are essential ones.

MEDICAL CANNABIS AND MARIJUANA

The amount of money and of legal energy being given to prosecute hundreds of thousands of Americans who are caught with a few ounces of marijuana in their jeans simply makes no sense— the kindest way to put it. A sterner way to put it is that it is an outrage, an imposition on basic civil liberties and on the reasonable expenditure of social energy.
—WILLIAM F. BUCKLEY

Today more than 50% of US states have medical cannabis laws, which give 80% of the US population potential access to medical cannabis. In some states, adults' personal use of marijuana is now legal. At the federal level, marijuana is still illegal, which has made research difficult and hindered its progress. (I use the term "cannabis" to refer to medical use and "marijuana" when referring to adult personal use.)

Originally all medications came from plants, and most of our modern medicines do too. Besides the opiates derived from the opium poppy, the medicines digitalis, penicillin, aspirin, quinine, vincristine, and many others originated in plants. Today's scientists are constantly looking at plant chemistry to find new medications.

One of these was the Chinese scientist Tu Youyou. She was awarded the Nobel Prize in 2015 for developing a new category of medicines, the main one being artemisinin. How did she come to discover these drugs? While studying ancient texts of traditional Chinese herbal medicine, she came across mention of sweet wormwood used to treat "intermittent fevers." Intermittent fevers are one of the hallmarks of malaria. She then set about isolating the active compounds and thus discovered new treatments. From these plants, she extracted artemisinin, which has helped millions of people worldwide.

Marijuana, too, has been used for thousands of years to treat a wide variety of ailments. Unfortunately, our country has a history of irrational marijuana phobia that is disproportionate to the drug's risks. I've read numerous studies and am convinced that there is a place for cannabis in helping patients. Yes, there are risks, as there are with just about every other medication. But when marijuana is used responsibly, its benefits clearly outweigh the risks.

> *The same drug that had been considered fearsome twenty years earlier, when associated with African Americans and Latinos, was refashioned as a relatively harmless drug when associated with whites.*
> —MICHELLE ALEXANDER, THE NEW JIM CROW:
> MASS INCARCERATION IN THE AGE OF COLORBLINDNESS

The federal government, through the Drug Enforcement Administration, classifies drugs with a risk of abuse. These classes are called Schedules 1 to 5, with 1 being the most dangerous. Schedule 1 includes substances alleged to have high risks and no proven benefits. This class includes heroin, LSD, psilocybin, and marijuana. Schedule 2 drugs are those with significant risks but also significant uses. Drugs in this class include the stronger opioids, amphetamines, and cocaine (used to stop bleeding and reduce pain in some surgeries). Schedule 3 drugs include milder opioids, like hydrocodone-acetaminophen (Lortab) and paracetamol-acetaminophen (Tylenol #3), and anabolic (bodybuilding) steroids that have other legitimate medical uses. Dronabinol (Marinol), a pill form of THC, which is the main active ingredient in marijuana, is listed under Schedule 3. Recently, the FDA (US Food and Drug Administration) has approved cannabis-based medicines for rare and severe epileptic conditions.

I find it inconsistent that marijuana is classified Schedule 1 while its main active ingredient is Schedule 3. Marinol has its uses, but it has numerous drawbacks as well. For example, it's hard to take a pill by mouth when nauseated. Once taken, the effect lasts for hours, which is not a benefit to those seeking quick relief. Its absorption rate in the body varies; therefore its effect can be unpredictable.

To round out the list, Schedule 4 includes the most common tranquilizers and sleeping pills like diazepam (Valium), and Schedule 5 includes very mild opioids, like those found in cough syrup or anti-diarrhea medicines.

Does marijuana belong in the same category with heroin and LSD? Most would agree that, although not completely free of risk, marijuana's risks are nowhere near as dangerous as the drugs with which it has been classed. One suggestion is that the DEA move marijuana from Schedule 1 to Schedule 3. The argument can also be made that cannabis ought not to be classified at all. However the needed change comes about, medical cannabis should be properly and consistently tested, measured, and dosed. Pharmaceutical companies, large and small, would enter the market and create standardized products that doctors could prescribe and pharmacists could dispense. Unfortunately, the War on Drugs in the United States led to categorizing marijuana a Schedule 1 drug, meaning that it has no medical use and is not safe. This irrational policy has halted or hampered cannabis research in this country for decades.

Fortunately, that was not the case elsewhere in the world. In Israel in the 1950s, a young scientist, Raphael Mechoulam, decided that he would study cannabis. Over years, Mechoulam identified its various active ingredients, such as THC and CBD (cannabidiol). He also surmised that for cannabinoid compounds to have an effect on humans, there must be cannabinoid receptors on cells in our body. After all, for a chemical to work biologically, it has to find a receptor. When you eat something, parsley, say, and nothing special happens, it either has no special chemical substance or we have no receptor for what it does have. Ingest an opioid, however, and the drug triggers receptors in the cells of our body. This insight that there must be receptors in our bodies on which opioids and other drugs act led to our understanding the endogenous endorphin system in the human body. Similarly, we now know that our bodies make endocannabinoids and that we have built-in cannabinoid chemistry. Otherwise, why would the receptors be there?

A critical difference between cannabis and opioids is that there are opioid receptors in the breathing center of our brain, but there are no cannabinoid receptors there. The intake of too much opioid shuts down the breathing center, and that's what leads to overdose deaths. Because there are no cannabinoid receptors in the brainstem, there have been no cannabis overdose deaths recorded in human history. Let me repeat that: no one has ever died from a cannabis overdose. That's not to say there aren't risk factors from cannabis, but stopping breathing or stopping your heart isn't among them.

No one has ever died from a cannabis overdose.

There's a medical term known as the "therapeutic index." It's a measure of the difference between a therapeutic dose of a medicine and its toxic dose. This is relevant for opioids and for many other medicines, such as anticoagulants, digoxin, and lithium (used to treat bipolar disorder), where the margin between treatment and overdose is narrow and thus the therapeutic index is low. But the therapeutic index for cannabis is essentially infinite, meaning that you can't die of a cannabis overdose. Feel sick? Possibly. Drop dead? No.

Polling shows that more than 80% of Americans favor medical cannabis. Rather than wait for the federal government to act, citizens lobbied at the state level. In response, some states took matters into their own hands and legalized medical cannabis use. There are also states that allow personal adult use, but let's stick to medical use for now.

This state-sponsored approach has moved things forward, but it has also led to a national patchwork of different laws. You'd have to check out your own state's laws to understand what your options are.

I remember one patient, many years ago, who changed my views on cannabis. She was an elderly woman who came to the ER for nausea and vomiting caused by a combination of bowel cancer and chemotherapy. After her condition improved a bit with medication and fluids, she grabbed me by the arm and wouldn't let go. "Doc," she said, as she held on, "Have you ever had real bad nausea? Ever been seasick? [Yes, I said.] Have you ever had food poisoning when you didn't know whether to sit on the toilet or put your head in it? [Yes.] When you were younger, did you ever drink too much and barf or wake up after with horrible stomach cramps? [Once in college.] I know you never had morning sickness, but did your wife? [Yes.] Well, doc, that's what I go through all the time. I'm fine and then a wave of nausea hits me, and the only thing that helps me right then is a puff of marijuana. I get quick relief, and I take enough for that but not enough to get stoned." We kept talking, just the two of us in the room. She explained that when the sickness struck, she was not able to take a pill or suppository; and even if she did, it took hours to work. I asked her where she got the marijuana, and she revealed that her son went out to buy it on the street, putting himself at risk. It was obvious that she was seeking medical help and was not a criminal. But under the laws of the time, she was. When I got to the legislature, I remembered her and resolved to do something about it.

In Maryland, like most other states, medical cannabis has been a bipartisan effort. Bills had been introduced before, but it was not until 2003 that the first bill passed. While it did not create a medical cannabis system, it did take a small step in the right direction by allowing for an "affirmative defense," meaning that a person caught with marijuana would not get a criminal penalty if the person could prove medical need.

In the years that followed, there were many attempts to get medical cannabis passed. With continued public pressure, over a period of 8 years (2010–2018), the medical cannabis program in Maryland was established. Our approach was not ideal. I would have structured much of it differently had I been able to. But politics is the art of the possible, and so compromises were made. Fortunately, Maryland now has a program that operates reasonably well. Included in it are research possibilities, which, I hope, will lead to medical progress.

During those years, people would tell me that I was politically courageous to introduce these bills. I didn't think so; it just made medical sense to me. The people who were courageous were the ones in Maryland and in other states who publicly testified— on the record, with their names and addresses documented—to using medical cannabis illegally. This testimony occurred in hearing rooms with police present. I was inspired by these ordinary responsible citizens who were willing to testify at great risk to themselves. These were the people who made medical cannabis programs possible in states across our country.

Many people testified before the Maryland state legislature at bill hearings to support medical cannabis. One was a 55-year-old chemist and mother of three, Kathy, who developed leukemia. Four years before giving her testimony, she underwent a bone marrow transplant at Johns Hopkins Hospital. After 60 days in isolation, struggling to take 17 medications per day, she grew progressively weaker and sicker. Such a downhill course is a known possibility for bone marrow transplant patients. When talking among themselves, medical professionals sometimes refer to this failing state of health as "circling the drain." The fear is that the cancer will be cured yet the patient nevertheless will die from the treatment and its side effects.

Everything had been tried to curb Kathy's nausea and increase her appetite, but she simply could not eat and was wasting away to skin and bones. Finally, the possibility of using marijuana was raised. Her Hopkins oncologist could only shrug: "I can't officially recommend it, but you can do whatever you feel you must."

Somehow marijuana was obtained, meaning that somebody bought it for her illegally. Without government oversight, of course, there was no way for Kathy to know for sure that the substance was genuine and not adulterated. Fortunately, in this case, it was the real product.

For 2 months Kathy smoked marijuana several times a week, just enough to stimulate her appetite and decrease her nausea but not enough to get significantly intoxicated. It worked. She gained weight and slowly recovered. Today, she's doing fine. She never used marijuana before or has since. She credits it with saving her life. Many other people told similar stories: a young man with cerebral palsy, a middle-aged man with post-polio pain syndrome, a young woman army veteran with multiple sclerosis. These people were not criminals, in my view, but to our judicial system they were.

Adolescent use of marijuana declined by 9% in states that allow adult personal use of marijuana.

Some may worry that liberalization of cannabis laws will lead to increased use by adolescents. Carefully conducted studies show, however, that the opposite has happened. A July 2019 article in JAMA *Pediatrics* reported that medical cannabis laws had no impact on adolescent use and that adolescent use had declined by 9% in states that allow adult personal use of marijuana. The reasons for this are not clear, but one of the authors speculated about it: "It may actually be more difficult for adolescents to obtain marijuana as drug dealers are replaced by licensed dispensaries that require proof of age. Selling to minors becomes a relatively more risky proposition after the passage of these laws."

As cannabis use becomes more widespread, we are learning more about it. One oncologist recommends it for his patients suffering from appetite loss, telling them to use the medication about 30 minutes before mealtime. He reports that his patients are responding well to this regimen.

There is some evidence that marijuana could be linked to the onset of schizophrenia in teenagers, but it's also possible that these young people are self-medicating to mask and manage their symptoms. Teen use, therefore, should be restricted to medical necessity.

Some chronic heavy users have developed marijuana hyperemesis syndrome, an uncommon condition characterized by repeated vomiting. This resolves when marijuana use is stopped.

There's no doubt that cannabis science is proceeding, but it will take years before we have a solid understanding of this amazing plant and its chemical derivatives. So far, over 60 cannabinoids have been identified, and of these only THC has psychoactive properties. The plant and all its derivatives need thorough study, and new strains with different properties are being developed.

We are learning about the endocannabinoid system: a complex chemical regulatory network within the human body. As with endorphins, our bodies make cannabinoids naturally. We are just beginning to understand this system, but it's widely involved in regulating many cellular activities, from brain function to the immune system.

There are numerous conditions for which cannabis can be helpful, and more are being investigated. The most commonly known ones are epilepsy and anorexia (loss of appetite). Cannabis may also be helpful for dysmenorrhea (menstrual cramps), Parkinson's disease, inflammatory bowel diseases (such as Crohn's disease), migraine headaches, sickle cell anemia pain, and side effects of cancer chemotherapy. Cannabinoid receptors have been found in bone cells; someday there may be a cannabinoid medicine that helps heal fractures.

Cannabis medicine can be taken in a variety of ways. This is a route of administration issue, much like any other medicine. For example, an anti-nausea medicine can be given by mouth, by injection, by patch, or as a rectal suppository. The route depends on the patient and their circumstances.

So too with cannabis. Very few patients are smoking raw buds in cigarette (joint) form. It can be harsh on the lungs, and smelly cannabis smoke is released (think of a Cheech and Chong movie). Cannabis for inhalation now comes in vaporizers, and these avoid the chemicals and smoke that come from combustion.

For a cancer patient suffering from chemo-induced nausea, an inhalational form of cannabis would be ideal. That might also work well for a woman with episodes of severe menstrual cramps. But for a child with epilepsy, a liquid form given by dropper under the tongue would be best. Someone with multiple sclerosis might do best with a long-acting oral dose titrated to relieve nerve pain and muscle spasms but not so much as to impair function. In other words, every patient is different and requires an individual treatment plan.

Our nation's approach to medical cannabis is irrational, unscientific, and harmful. Furthermore, as other nations advance their cannabis research, our scientists are left behind. Yes, I wish cannabis could go through all the formal testing required by the FDA. But waiting for that to happen and for federal policy to change would take decades. That won't help the people who are suffering now, and that's why I support medical cannabis.

Research is now under way into the uses of another Schedule 1 drug: psilocybin. Preliminary data suggests that it can greatly benefit those with serious or terminal illnesses when used under carefully controlled conditions. (See the Resources section for suggested reading on this topic.)

For those with advanced illness and approaching the end of life, cannabis can bring special benefit. Somatic symptoms, such as loss of appetite, can be helped. On its own or combined with other medicines, cannabis can help relieve anxiety, pain, and muscle spasms. There is no need to worry about long-term consequences. Cannabis can also be a mood elevator and make people feel better. Is there anything wrong with a person with advanced illness getting a little high?

Many patients have told me that it is not death they fear but the pain that may come in dying. Pain can and should be treated. There have been unfortunate instances of narcotics, opioids, or cannabis being withheld out of fear of producing an addiction, even when the potential addict has only months or weeks to live. Physicians and patients should maintain an open dialogue about the best ways to relieve pain and other symptoms that interfere with quality of life. As the patient's condition changes, so might their choices.

But there is one thing we should all agree on: In the War on Drugs, isn't it time to take the sick and dying off the battlefield? People in pain should not be held hostage to an irrational political agenda.

> *In order to rise from its own ashes,*
> *a Phoenix first must burn.*
> —OCTAVIA BUTLER

10

What's Stopping Us

*Die? I should say not, dear fellow. No Barrymore would
allow such a conventional thing to happen to him.*
—John Barrymore

WHY DON'T MORE AMERICANS COMPLETE
ADVANCE DIRECTIVES?

How many Americans have an advance directive? This question
arose as I worked on public policy questions in the Maryland legislature relating to end-of-life care. I assumed it would be an easy
question to answer. A "cohort," in public health terms, refers to a
group of people with the same or a similar medical condition, for
example, those with kidney cancer or sickle cell anemia. I can look
up and easily find out how many people there are in these cohorts
and any number of other conditions.

Death, of course, is the cohort to which we all will eventually
belong. With the economics being what they are, I assumed that
key organizations such as the American Public Health Association
would address this. I reviewed the association's website (www
.apha.org), where there's a long list of its priority issues. The list includes the items you'd expect (and maybe some you wouldn't), and
they are the standard and important ones: climate change, mental

health, gun violence, maternal and child health, substance misuse, suicide, tobacco, communicable diseases, and vaccinations, among others. End-of-life care? Not there.

I thought this would have made the list, but I was wrong.

I got in touch with the association and asked about end-of-life care. I was told that the association didn't consider this to be a public health issue, which I was surprised to learn about this key organization. Although our public institutions collect data on almost every facet of health care, this is one area where data was scarce.

> *The taboo against talking about death may explain why a key public health organization does not make end-of-life care one of its priorities.*

Why don't public health organizations look at this? While I have no proof, my guess is that it reflects our culture's aversion to anything related to death and dying. That taboo is so strong that the groups able to tackle virtually every other pressing public health matter have avoided this one.

Meanwhile my question of how many Americans have completed advance directives remained unanswered. I decided that since no one else was doing the research, I would.

My colleague Professor Keshia Pollack Porter, at the Johns Hopkins Bloomberg School of Public Health, and I designed a study to investigate the rate of completion of advance directives and people's attitudes toward them ("Public Perspectives on Advance Directives: Implications for State Legislative and Regulatory Policy," *Health Policy*, February 2010; and "End-of-Life Care Issues: A Personal, Economic, Public Policy, and Public Health Crisis," *American Journal of Public Health*, April 18, 2013).

Our study included a sophisticated survey with follow-up analysis. We focused on Maryland, but because Maryland's population demographics mirror those of the United States, what we learned has broad application nationally. We discovered a number of interesting things.

Our research revealed that while only about a third of Americans had completed an advance directive, more than 80% of people over age 18 wanted their end-of-life wishes to be respected. This finding identified a significant gap: people had given thought to the question of their end-of-life care, but the majority hadn't completed the forms that would direct it.

Why didn't people complete advance directives? About a quarter of the respondents said they didn't know about them. Others felt that they were too young or healthy to need them, or they were concerned about the cost, the complexity of the questions, or the time that might be required to complete them.

Age was a significant factor. Younger people were much less likely than older people to have filled out an advance directive. It may seem unnecessary for a younger person to have such a document, but as we saw earlier, the three most famous cases in American legal history concerning end-of-life care all involved people under the age of 30: Karen Ann Quinlan, Nancy Cruzan, and Terri Schiavo. Had these young women prepared advance directives, much heartache and legal hostility would probably have been avoided.

Americans are concerned about their end-of-life care and want to be involved in it, but most don't complete the forms that plan for that care.

We asked people where they would prefer to get information about advance directives. Overwhelmingly, they wanted to obtain it from their doctors or other health care providers, rather than from attorneys, clergy, or online sources. While younger people, not surprisingly, were more comfortable locating information on the internet, nearly everyone wanted the opportunity to review their decisions with medical professionals. This finding means that doctors, nurses, and health care personnel of all types have an important role to play.

Our study demonstrated that Americans are concerned about end-of-life care, and they want to be involved. We need to increase the public's awareness of how important these issues are and provide better information about them.

MINORITY AND DIVERSITY PERSPECTIVES

We also identified diversity issues. Our country is made up of many different types of people with a wide range of spiritual and cultural backgrounds. As a physician, I've always done my best to work with each patient personally, but I know at times I've come up short. Try as I might, the reality is that I can't relate perfectly to everyone, and sometimes the problems are based not on any ill will but rather on the difficulty of bridging differences in background, especially in an emergency room setting. That's why, again, it's important to address these issues in advance.

From our analysis of the rate of completion of advance directives, Keshia and I reported that the rate among minorities was lower than in the white population. We wrote,

> About twice as many Whites as African Americans completed advance directives. The difference between Whites and African Americans regarding the prevalence of advance directives is likely attributable to several factors, including cultural differences in family-centered decision-making, distrust of the health care system, or poor communication between health care professionals and patients. Research in other areas suggests that African Americans prefer to involve multiple family members, friends, and clergy in making health care decisions. Thus, they may be more likely to designate a health care agent to coordinate that decision-making rather than state their own preferences in a living will.

We can speculate on the reasons for this. Historical events have left their scars. Minorities have a distrust of the health care system.

In the Tuskegee experiment (1930–1972) 600 African American men were offered free medical care, but instead they were left untreated for syphilis, even after penicillin cures had become available, so that the disease's natural history could be studied. In the 1950s, cells from a tumor from Henrietta Lacks were harvested by the Johns Hopkins Hospital. These cells became the basis of major research experiments, but neither the patient nor her family were ever informed about this. Charles Drew was a physician and researcher who developed much of the science behind blood transfusion procedures and testing. He fought the Red Cross policy that maintained racial segregation in blood donation until 1950.

There's a long history in the United States of unequal health care based on race.

There are too many examples of African Americans and other minorities receiving substandard care. An examination of this history of unequal treatment is well summarized in the *New York Times'* podcast 1619 in the episode "Bad Blood." The episode opens with a heartbreaking story of a person whose care was so delayed that he died of what would have been a treatable cancer. Tragically, this story is all too common.

This history, along with daily shortfalls in the quality and availability of health care, has left many minority groups worried about end-of-life care. To state it plainly, their concern is that the health care system will expedite the deaths of minority patients. Some have even told me they worry that the plug will be pulled early so that organs can be harvested for white people.

I've done many presentations in churches and other settings with a largely minority audience. I make the case that advance directives are a tool of empowerment and one of the best ways to increase the likelihood that you'll get the care you want. At some of these, I've been joined by my friend Aquanetta Betts, who is an estate planning attorney. Together, we've motivated many people to get their medical and financial paperwork in order. Given the power and influence of churches, and indeed all religious institutions, I hope that more of these will bring this topic to the attention of their congregants.

There are cultural norms, but there is also a great diversity of values and personalities within each community. We should be careful not to stereotype anyone based on their background.

I worked for limited stints several times on a Navajo Indian Reservation in Chinle, Arizona. My job was covering ER shifts over the June–July annual staff transition period. The Navajo approach to end-of-life care was different from anything I was used to, so I had to adapt. For example, the Navajo way is to bury the dead as soon as possible. Navajos also prefer that a dying person not die at home and instead be taken to another location or a hospital to die. Burying the deceased involves another set of rules and rituals.

Learning about how other cultures approach death reshaped my own thinking about it.

Learning about how other cultures approach death and the words they use to talk about it has reshaped my own thinking. There's a Native American term for dying that I came across while reading a local newspaper in a small Oregon town. Obituaries in that paper described the person who died as having "walked on." Swahili culture uses the terms "sasha" and "zamani." "Sasha" refers to those who have died and were known personally to people currently alive. "Zamani" refers to the spirits of people in the distant past who are no longer personally known to the living. This struck me as an intriguing way to think about time and recollection.

Many hospices are now reaching out to minority communities and are actively recruiting minority physicians and nurses to help spread the word that hospice is about quality of life and that its use should be increased.

Having a more diverse health care team helps. Sadly, prejudices still exist, and we are all to some extent influenced by our own biases. On a few occasions, I've seen white patients not want to be taken care of by a person of color. These few episodes took place many years ago, but it's made me wonder how often that feeling is there but unstated. Likewise, I've wondered whether some of my patients of color would have been more comfortable under the care of someone who looked more like them than I do. It's not just race; it can be age or gender too. Some clinicians are uncomfortable with teenagers or with very old people.

I remember an episode at the Navajo hospital when I was taking care of an 8-year-old boy who had been thrown from a horse and sustained a fracture to his leg. I was explaining to the parents that he would need to be transferred to another hospital for definitive care. They were staring at me blankly, saying, "Don't tell us. Tell him." I was used to talking with parents about their child's medical condition, but in the Navajo culture, the clinician addresses the child directly along with the parents. So I shifted my focus, and everyone was more comfortable.

Hopefully, our health care workforce at all levels will eventually reflect the diversity of our population, and these barriers can be minimized.

COMPASSIONOMICS

It's important that health care providers make clear that they care about their patients and not just because it's a nice thing to do. Recent studies have shown that demonstrating even a minute (40 to 60 seconds) of compassion has beneficial effects. Patients do better. It also turns out that compassion is a two-way street because providers experience less burnout. This new approach is called "compassionomics," and its pioneers are physicians Anthony Mazzarelli and Stephen Trzeciak. Check out their research and Trzeciak's TED Talk (see Resources).

I've long tried to bring this to my work as an ER doctor. For example, if possible, I try to sit down after I first meet the patient rather than stay standing. This brings a sense of presence. I try not to interrupt when a patient is telling me about their problem, at least not for the first 2 to 3 minutes. You'd be surprised how hard that can be. If there are other people in the room with the patient, I always ask their names and their connection to the patient.

Compassion matters for patients and for care providers.

Doing these things builds a personal connection, not easy to do in a busy ER, but it's well worth the few extra seconds it takes.

Compassionomics takes this to a new level, one based on data, and it ought to be applied by all health care providers in all settings. In fact, perhaps it ought to be included in other interactions too: lawyers with clients, bosses with employees, teachers with students, police with citizens, and so on.

Practicing compassionomics might also ease some of the diversity communication challenges I mentioned above. If we know someone actually cares about us, our defenses tend to relax, and a better, more productive engagement can follow.

WAYS TO BRING THE SUBJECT UP

We've made some progress, but more research is needed to answer the key question: What can be done to motivate more Americans, across all demographics, to complete advance directives and, where appropriate, MOLST/POLST?

Talking about advance directives needs to become a routine part of doctor-patient conversations so that the topic becomes "normalized." The more routine the topic becomes, the less scary it is. The reality, unfortunately, is that the subject of advance directives is not yet part of most medical exams. It's not even generally included as part of a patient's electronic health record, although medications, blood pressure recordings, and allergies are. Until such time that it is, we must be the ones to take care of this issue for ourselves and our loved ones.

Every so often, an end-of-life care story gets media attention. The case of Terri Schiavo in 2004–2005 led to a surge in requests for advance directives. Since then, requests for advance directives have quieted down.

Let's say you've moved beyond the initial discomfort everyone feels about end-of-life issues. What if you want to open the discussion with your spouse, a family member, or a friend? Many people are in denial on this subject. If you try to bring it up, they may shrug off your attempt with a joke or a rebuff. Physicians and nurses are not immune to denial, either. When this topic came up in a conversation I had with a friend who's a surgeon, he just grimaced and replied, "It'll all work out somehow or other." While what he said is undeniably true, the way it will work out may not be to his liking. Even with as much experience as he's had with illness and dying, he was simply unwilling to face the fact of his own eventual death.

One way to raise the topic is to make it part of a shared exercise. Aging with Dignity, the organization behind the "Five Wishes" format for advance directives, suggests hosting a Five Wishes party. Invite all the adult members of your family plus any other interested friends and give a copy of the Five Wishes document to everyone. A gathering like this gives people the chance to ask questions, talk over the issues involved in choosing a health care agent, and explore the level of care they would prefer for themselves in different situations. Aging with Dignity provides an instructional DVD, called *Sharing the Gift*, and a facilitator's guide that can be used to prepare the group for filling out the forms. The Conversation Project is another online resource that facilitates end-of-life care discussions.

Benjamin Franklin wrote, "Nothing can be said to be certain, except death and taxes." Playing on this wisdom, National Healthcare Decisions Day (NHDD) comes around every April 16. It's easy to remember since it comes right after Tax Day on April 15. Many states and localities recognize NHDD, which prompts people to complete or review their advance directive.

Whether or not you use these resources, it's helpful to complete advance directives together with your family and friends. When you invite people to such a gathering, be sure to have the relevant forms available. Either fill out your own advance directive at the same time as everyone else or bring your already completed advance directive with you for the others to read if you are willing to share it. At the very least, you can discuss your own experience in completing the form. Some people may want to have more time to consider the questions raised by an advance directive; in that case, you can schedule a follow-up meeting.

Persistence pays off. You never can quite know what words or events will finally move someone to action. Even if you get negative or passive responses at first, continue to bring up the subject from time to time. As my and Keshia's research showed, people want to take care of this kind of advance planning. Many of them just need someone to break the ice. That person can be you.

We must build dikes of courage to hold back the flood of fear.
—MARTIN LUTHER KING JR.

11

Gifts of Life

ORGAN DONATION, FUNERALS, AND CEMETERIES

———

I think you should automatically donate your organs because that would turn the balance of organ donation in a huge way. I would donate whatever anybody would take.
—George Clooney

ADVANCE DIRECTIVES AND ORGAN DONATION

To review: The first part of an advance directive designates the kind and degree of care you wish to receive. This can be supplemented by MOLST/POLST forms. The second part specifies the people you choose as your health care decision makers.

The third part of the advance directive addresses a variety of related issues: organ donation, funeral plans, and body disposition.

THE US ORGAN DONATION SYSTEM

The bumper sticker says it all: "Don't take your organs to heaven. We need them right here on earth."

The science of organ donation has advanced rapidly over the past 10 to 20 years. Every year organ transplantation helps thousands of people live longer and more productive lives. Still, more than 115,000 Americans are waiting for organs, and it's estimated that about 25 people on the waiting list die each day.

Don't take your organs to heaven. We need them right here on earth.

For organ donation, there are three categories of tissues that can be used. The first comes from people who are recently dead. These are known as cadaver donations. These tissues include skin (used for burns), bones and tendons (for orthopedic repairs), and the cornea of the eye (for replacing damaged ones).

The second category comes from people who are alive and healthy. Since we are born with two kidneys, it is possible to donate one and still lead a normal life. The same is true of a bone marrow donation or a portion of the lobe of one's liver. Usually the donor needs to be a genetic match with the recipient.

The third category includes vital organs like the heart and lungs. These come from people on life support with no hope of recovery, and the donors will die immediately after the organs are removed. That's why the determination of brain death for them is so important.

Almost all advance directive forms include a section relating to organ donation. Within this, there are several choices. One can specify that only certain organs be taken, such as skin or corneas, or that all usable organs can be transplanted. One donor can help many others with their tissues.

When I started as an ER doctor, it fell to me to ask families about organ donation for their deceased relative. Frankly, there wasn't any training. Patients and families had many questions, and I didn't have all the answers, nor did I have the time to sit with families and discuss the options. I did the best I could and was often able to get consent for corneal donations. But then organ donation science was in its infancy, and there wasn't too much to ask for. As transplant science became more complex and as new diseases appeared (like HIV/AIDS), the questions became harder and the discussions longer, and I honestly was not equipped to do a good job. To do that well takes special training and focus. Fortunately, this situation has improved.

There are now national standards, but the details of transplant law are determined by state governments. When I got to the state legislature, I worked to update and improve the laws in Maryland. It wasn't easy, as there were many issues to be worked out, from religious concerns to financial ones. Fortunately, several organ donation groups banded together and provided solid information, and these concerns were addressed.

The most effective testimony, as always, came from people personally affected. I'll never forget those hearings. These were people whose lives were saved by donated organs. They had received kidneys, hearts, livers, lungs. They were alive because someone had given them the "gift of life," as organ donation is known. Also present in support were the families of donors. They testified that they had received solace knowing their loved one helped someone else live. These hearings went on for hours. Tears were shed by the families of both recipients and donors. All the legislators and those in the audience (often there for other bills on the agenda) got misty-eyed as well. It was impossible not to be touched. Thankfully, my 2008 bill written to reform our system was passed. The new law created one organization that coordinates an organ donation registry and organ collection statewide.

On a national basis, the country is divided into regions determined by the Centers for Medicare and Medicaid Services, known as CMS (not a typo; there's only one "M" in the abbreviation). CMS certifies and regulates organ procurement organizations (OPOs), and there is one OPO for each region. All OPOs are nonprofit.

The OPOs work together through data sharing, managed by the United Network for Organ Sharing (UNOS), a national non-profit organization created by the US Congress. UNOS promotes scientific and educational efforts, and it sets policies to ensure that organ donation is handled fairly and appropriately. UNOS is there to coordinate, say, if a kidney available in Texas genetically matches a patient in Maine so that arrangements can be made. We are fortunate in the United States to have a national system.

The trained staff of an OPO come to wherever they are needed, usually to an ER or intensive care unit. The on-site medical providers play an important role by starting the conversation with family members and by identifying possible donors early on and contacting the local OPO. Getting the OPO active early gives more time for thought and discussion and for making sure that everything is in order. The OPO staff then manage all the organ donation issues. They have the skills and the time to provide fully informed answers to questions. I'll try to answer the most common questions about organ donation here, but the conversation between the patient (or their health care agent) and the transplant expert will be central to decision-making.

Q: Does it cost money to donate an organ?
A: No, there is no cost.

Q: What if the deceased has an illness or other condition?
A: Each case is assessed individually. Even people who die of cancer can be donors.

Q: Are there age limits?
A: No. A person of any age can be a donor.

Q: I'm not sure if my religion supports organ donation.
A: Almost all major religions do support organ donation, and information is available for each.

Q: What if I'm near death? Will the medical staff not save me in order to get my organs?

A: The medical staff's first priority is your well-being. Donation is not considered until all medical care is deemed futile.

Q: How will my organs be distributed?

A: There are state and national databases that match organs to potential recipients fairly.

Q: Could someone take my organs and sell them?

A: No. It's against US law and medical ethics. All organ donations are closely monitored.

Q: Does a donation make an open casket impossible?

A: No. All organs can be removed without disturbing the appearance of the deceased for an open-casket funeral service.

The OPO arranges the testing for biological and genetic compatibility (known as an HLA profile), and that information is entered into a national database so that matches can be established.

What is key to all this is that people sign up to be organ donors. Doing so is quick and easy through Donate Life America (www.donatelife.net), and there are state chapters as well. You can sign up for both the national and state registries, and the website provides useful information on all aspects of organ donation. All your information is protected and shared only between Donate Life and your regional OPO. As with advance directives, you can change your mind about organ donation at any time.

Decisions about organ donation do not have to be part of an advance directive, but it's best if they are. Notation on a driver's license is helpful, but it does not go into specifics about what organs are to be used. However one's donor status is documented, experts review the patient's wishes and medical condition and discuss organ donation with family members.

A dear friend of mine was the mother of a 19-year-old man who died of a head injury in a sudden tragic accident. She spoke at her son's memorial service. Others had preceded her and told stories of his life, but she spoke briefly to share the following: "When my son was 16 and got his driver's license, he had no hesitation in designating himself as an organ donor. Today I received a letter that two people can now see because of corneal transplants, and 50 more are helped by his skin, bones, and tendons. And there are others whose lives were saved by his heart, lungs, pancreas, liver, and kidneys. Yes, he is gone, but not only does his memory live on; it gives us great comfort to know that the gift of his body gives life to others."

During the bill hearings, there was another aspect of organ donation that was amazing to see. If both a recipient and a donor's family want to meet, the OPO can arrange an introduction. Several pairs of these folks told their stories, sitting next to each other at the witness table. It was incredible to see a family hugging a person who now had the heart of their child.

My recommendation? Sign up to be an organ donor.

WHAT IS BRAIN DEATH?

How do we know when someone is actually dead? At first glance, this would seem obvious. As someone who has declared people dead in the ER, I never had any doubt about it, and I am not aware of any instance where someone was declared dead and turned out to be alive.

How do we know when someone is dead?

There are the obvious cases: someone with a traumatic head injury. In the ER I've seen that with gunshot wounds to the head or with a motorcycle rider who had not worn a helmet. Then there are those not revived after prolonged CPR. For the latter, there are now new techniques that document the failure of the heart to beat, such as bedside ultrasound showing no cardiac activity.

There are some situations when it is important not to declare someone dead too quickly. The most common one is when the person has a low body temperature, known as hypothermia, which can occur in a cold-water drowning. Sometimes the lower body temperature protects against brain damage, and there have been many cases where a person fell through the ice into cold water, was underwater for a prolonged time, yet was later revived with minimal residual damage or even a full recovery. In those cases, the person is warmed to normal body temperature before any decisions are made, and sometimes that can take hours. A saying in the ER is that a person has to be both "warm and dead" before a final determination is made.

With the development of ventilators, new medicines, and the latest techniques, people's bodies can be kept alive for long periods of time. Years, in fact. It used to be thought that when the brain died, so did the rest of the body. But now people who are declared brain dead are sometimes sustained long enough for their bodies to heal or even to grow, although the ultimate outcome never changes. The central question then becomes, When is a person "brain dead"? That is, when has an irreversible coma set in with no hope of recovery?

Sometimes families pray for a miracle recovery and hope that a person in an irreversible coma will wake up. However, a 2018 article from the *Journal of the American Medical Association* stated, "Brain death represents a state of very severe neurological injury with no evidence, to date, that anyone correctly diagnosed will ever regain consciousness or breathe without a ventilator."

The key then is to make sure the patient is correctly diagnosed, and criteria for this have been developed and are provided in the Uniform Determination of Death Act (UDDA), which all 50 states have adopted. There are two main uses for the UDDA.

The first is that it helps families understand why prolonging life-sustaining treatments may be stopped. Knowing this relieves them of the anxiety and guilt of ending care. The second is to facilitate organ donation.

WHOLE BODY DONATION

Some people arrange to donate their bodies to scientific research and medical education. Bodies donated to medical schools help physicians-in-training and other health care professionals learn human anatomy. The anatomy lab is an important class taken early in medical school. Without donated bodies, it would be difficult, if not impossible, for doctors to gain a comprehensive understanding of human anatomy in all its beauty and complexity.

In my anatomy class, we spent 2 months working in teams, slowly dissecting and studying the human body. It was challenging at first, but over time we came to a deep appreciation for the knowledge we were gaining. And studying real bodies was truly the best and only way to get it. Anatomy lab instructors pass on to students the tradition of treating the donated bodies with respect. One friend told me that on her first day of anatomy class, the instructor warned the students that any wisecracks would result in dismissal from the class and an automatic "F."

For some people the idea of whole body donation seems ghoulish. For others, there is comfort in knowing that their bodies are helping others to learn. If you choose to donate your body to medical science, you'll need to make arrangements in advance with a medical school or state anatomy board. There is no cost incurred by these donations.

My mother donated her body to the medical school of UCLA (University of California, Los Angeles). She died in a fall at home. Because it was an unwitnessed event, the police were notified. After the coroner determined that her death was an accident, the UCLA team removed her body and transported it.

Shelley and I were in Los Angeles a year later, and we got an invitation from UCLA to attend a service for the families of people who had donated their bodies. We didn't know what to expect, but we went along with our daughter Sarah. Sarah lived in Los Angeles, and she and her grandmother had been close.

The service was lovely. The first-year medical students officiated, and they were all in attendance wearing white coats. They thanked us for the gift our relatives had provided, and it reminded me that this was how I, too, had learned human anatomy. Even with the best computer graphics and modeling, there is simply no substitute for dissection in the education of future physicians. Several of the students played music and shared poetry. A few told how this experience was shaping their medical career. Afterwards there was a reception, and each of us was given a flower to take home. About 200 family members were present, and it struck me what a diverse group we were. Some looked like they could be wealthy; others seemed of more modest means. The spectrum of races was a reflection of the different people who live in Los Angeles. I wish I could have talked more to everyone there to get insight into how their loved one came to the decision to donate, and how they felt about it. The entire event was gracious, respectful, and moving, and it made us appreciate my mother's choice.

I learned later that many medical schools hold similar events. If there are ones that don't, I suggest they look into inaugurating this tradition.

BODY DISPOSITION

Embalming, v.t.: To cheat vegetation by locking up the gases upon which it feeds. By embalming their dead and thereby deranging the natural balance between animal and vegetable life, the Egyptians made their once fertile and populous country barren and incapable of supporting more than a meagre crew. The modern metallic

burial casket is a step in the same direction, and many a dead man
who ought now to be ornamenting his neighbor's lawn as a tree,
or enriching his table as a bunch of radishes, is doomed to long
inutility. We shall get him after a while if we are spared, but in the
meantime the violet and rose are languishing for a nibble at his
gluteus maximus.
—AMBROSE BIERCE, THE DEVIL'S DICTIONARY

After we die, our bodies must go somewhere. Some people include instructions for what they want to happen to their earthly remains as part of their advance directives. There are options, depending on your beliefs, preferences, traditions, and means.

Most Americans choose to have a funeral home handle and dispose of their remains, either by burial or cremation. Prices vary, but today the average American funeral and burial costs between $8,000 and $10,000; some cost much more. Cremations range from $1,500 to $5,000, not including any costs of disposing of the cremated remains in a burial vault or a cemetery plot. Too many Americans can't afford these services, so they finance the cost and worsen their debt. Furthermore, families are vulnerable at these times. When someone beloved has just died, it's hard to think rationally about financial matters. Funeral directors provide a service, but they are also there to sell products. So they have a tendency to push items for sale or add surcharges for services that aren't necessary.

Often embalming is suggested. It's not required or needed, except perhaps when there is an extended delay between death and burial, such as when a person dies far from home and must be transported back. The embalming procedure drains all blood and fluids from the body and replaces these with formaldehyde. Morticians and casket makers experience higher-than-normal cancer rates caused by the toxic chemicals in embalming fluid and the finishes used on most coffins. These same chemicals go into the ground, along with the metal or hardwood coffins chosen by most

Americans. In addition, almost all US cemeteries require that the casket be interred in a concrete vault. This is not legally required, but it eases landscape maintenance. These are some of the environmental issues connected with standard funeral options.

THE DOWNSIDES OF EMBALMING AND CREMATION

According to the Casket and Funeral Association of America, each year in the United States, cemetery burials inter 827,000 gallons of embalming fluid and caskets containing 92,000 tons of steel, 2,700 tons of copper and bronze, and more than 30 million board-feet of hardwoods. Burial vaults consume 1,640,000 tons of reinforced concrete and 14,000 tons of steel. Once these materials are buried, they can no longer be reused or recycled. To look at these numbers in a different way, as Mark Harris wrote in his book *Grave Matters*: "The amount of wood from coffins in a ten-acre cemetery is enough to build 40 houses, and there's enough concrete to build swimming pools for all of them."

While some may think that cremation is an environmentally sound alternative, that is not the case. Cremation also has serious environmental drawbacks. It releases carbon dioxide, sulfur dioxide, and other greenhouse gases and persistent organic pollutants into the atmosphere. Each cremation uses the energy equivalent of 28 gallons of fuel and releases 540 pounds of carbon dioxide into the air, along with trace amounts of other harmful chemicals such as carbon monoxide and mercury.

Did you know that in most states there is no legal requirement to use a funeral home at all? A hundred years ago, when a person died, that person often was laid out at home in a living room or in the bedroom where the death had taken place. Visitors paid their respects, and the person was buried in the local burial ground or family plot behind the house. Today this tradition is no longer common, but it is still legal in almost every state. Once a proper death certificate is obtained, families can make their own arrangements for disposition of the body without the services of a funeral home. The laws and regulations for this vary from locality to locality. If this approach interests you, you should investigate the statutes and regulations where you live. More information about home funerals can be obtained from the National Home Funeral Alliance (www.homefuneralalliance.org).

There is a growing movement to return to natural burial practices, either in the "green" sections of established cemeteries or in new, natural burial preserves. There are now eco-friendly burial caskets on the market. This can be the traditional plain-wood casket or ones made from other natural materials, such as banana leaves or woven fibers, which degrade over time in a natural way. These are almost always less expensive than standard caskets.

In my first years in the Maryland state legislature, constituents sometimes called me months after a family member had been buried. In retrospect they realized how much more they had paid than they had wanted or expected to. One man, a carpenter, told he that he wanted to build a casket for his mother, but he was told that was not permitted under Maryland law. I checked, and he was right. At that time, only funeral directors could sell caskets. Caskets, I thought, are really only furniture; and if someone could build one, then they ought to be able to use it or sell it. I introduced legislation that changed this absurd restriction, and now caskets in Maryland can be made and sold by anyone.

NATURAL BURIAL

Citing spiritual, financial, and environmental reasons, more Americans are forgoing embalming and expensive caskets and opting instead for simpler and more natural ways to return their physical remains to the earth.

The first natural burial ground in the United States was Ramsey Creek Preserve in Westminster, South Carolina. It was started by Bill and Kimberly Campbell, and it has now grown to 71 acres, with over 1,500 burial sites. Embalming is not allowed, and all caskets must be simple and biodegradable. Shelley and I toured Ramsey Creek, and it is a beautiful preserved forest and meadowland. Walking around, here and there, you come across a flat fieldstone engraved with the name of someone deceased.

Natural burial is an environmentally sound option for returning the body to the earth in a simple and dignified way.

There are benches and rest areas throughout, allowing for contemplation and reflection. A nondenominational chapel is available for services. We found it more comforting than standard cemeteries, with their putting-green lawns, monuments laid out in rows, and a sense that those with larger monuments were more important than others with smaller ones.

Natural burial grounds also answer an important land-use question. How can undeveloped land be made affordable or even profitable without paving it or farming it or developing it into houses or businesses? In this case, the land pays for itself (taxes, upkeep, etc.) while keeping its pristine features: trees, birds, streams, and bushes. Today there are more than 90 American cemeteries across the country that offer natural burial. I suggest you check them out before making a disposition decision (www.greenburialcouncil .org).

Whatever method you choose for disposing of your body or the body of a loved one, survivors usually find comfort in a formal ceremony of remembrance. Whether at a solemn funeral mass in a house of worship or at a simple memorial service at home, friends and family have the opportunity to remember the deceased and say goodbye. Every religious faith has traditions about such commemorations. While some people feel that these ceremonies are not needed in our modern scientific world, I believe we should not disregard the collective psychological wisdom of the human race. Once death has occurred, our primary focus turns to bringing comfort to the survivors.

> The Kikuyu, when left to themselves, do not bury their dead, but leave them above ground for the hyenas and vultures to deal with. The custom had always appealed to me. I thought that it would be a pleasant thing to be laid out to the sun and the stars, and to be so promptly, neatly, and openly picked and cleansed; to be made one with Nature and become a common component of a landscape.
> —KAREN BLIXEN, OUT OF AFRICA

12

No Job Is Complete Until the Paperwork Is Done

MAKING IT LEGAL

———

The sweetest joy, the wildest woe is love. What the world really needs is more love and less paperwork.
—Pearl Bailey

We can lick gravity, but sometimes the paperwork is overwhelming.
—Wernher von Braun

MAKING IT LEGAL

For end-of-life planning to work, there are three key steps. First, you have to complete your advance directive, something only you can do. Second, it has to be available if and when needed. Last, health professionals need to understand and honor these forms.

There are challenges with each of these steps, but as the public becomes more interested in advance directives and the rate of completing the forms increases, these difficulties will diminish.

For an advance directive to be valid, a person needs to sign and date the form. The stipulations for the signature process vary from state to state, but the guiding principles are the same. Most states require that one or two other adults witness the person sign the form and attest it by adding their own signatures. A witness can be almost anyone: a friend, a coworker, a neighbor. A witness doesn't need to review the contents of your advance directive; a witness needs only to see you sign the form. Because of the increased popularity of online systems, many states now accept electronic witnessing. The only people who should *not* serve as witnesses are the persons designated to be your health care agents and anyone who stands to gain by your death through inheritance or as an insurance beneficiary. In addition, most states prohibit your health care provider from acting as a witness. These rules help ensure the neutrality of the witnesses and protect a vulnerable patient from being coerced by someone who could benefit from that individual's death.

You don't need an attorney to complete an advance directive.

In most states the witnesses must attest to knowing the individual personally and to believing the person to be of sound mind. In some states the signatures must be notarized by a notary public. Notaries can be found in the phone book or on the internet, and your bank or your lawyer may have a notary on staff. The Resources section of this book contains information about obtaining an advance directive form appropriate for your state.

You don't need an attorney to draft and authorize an advance directive. In fact, the forms are designed to be completed without legal advice. But if you want a lawyer to help you fill out the form, there are a variety of resources. These include AARP (American Association of Retired Persons), state attorney general offices, legal aid organizations, and private attorneys.

Copies of your advance directive should be kept in several locations: your doctor's office, your medical record, with your loved ones, and with whomever you have designated your health care agent. You should carry a copy (or a reduced-size version) with

How can you make your advance directive available when you are traveling?

you when you travel. Unlike other important documents, don't keep your advance directive locked up in a safe or a bank safe deposit box, or hidden in a file. It needs to be readily available when needed.

What happens if you get sick while you are traveling? Or if you are taken to a hospital where you don't usually get care? How will your advance directive be found? These are real concerns, but there are solutions.

ONLINE SYSTEMS: MYDIRECTIVES AND OTHERS

There are national registry systems. My personal favorite is MyDirectives.com, and it's the one I use. You begin by registering with your name and a password. The forms are clear, easy to use, and have helpful links that explain medical procedures if you are not familiar with them. You can enter details about any health issues, insurance, and contact information.

In addition to the standard required items, the MyDirectives website includes other areas where you can upload a video with a message to your doctor or family. You can specify other items, such as personal care or activity preferences. Periodically the system sends an alert reminding you to update the form if your health, relationships, circumstances, or wishes have changed.

We live in a mobile society and are not always close to our homes or regular health care systems. MyDirectives offers a QR code (a type of bar code) that contains your advance directive information. This can be printed as a wallet card or downloaded to your phone. The QR code can be read by medical personnel with a QR app reader, available for cell phones (figures 12.1 and 12.2).

Most smart phones have a medical ID application with which

you can link to your online advance directive, in addition to other important data. These documents are accessible even without the phone's passcode. Be sure to activate that app and provide the required information.

Another online source of advance directives is CAKE (www .joincake.com). The name "CAKE" suggests that you can have your cake and eat it too. Like MyDirectives, it walks you through aspects of end-of-life care planning, including, for example, assessing the need for life insurance, complete with links to various life insurance companies. CAKE also provides links to each state's standard advance directive form. With the CAKE system, you can upload forms that you've completed from other sources.

Both MyDirectives and CAKE work well and are free. There are likely new services becoming available.

Several states offer an advance directive registry to their residents. On a voluntary basis, residents can file their advance directive with the state's registry, where it is kept confidential and can only be accessed by appropriate persons. I believe that every state should make this service available.

I'm often asked what happens if you are traveling in another state when you need your advance directive. Will your advance directive be legally binding? There is no easy answer to that question. If you happen to spend a lot of time in two states, I suggest completing the advance directive for both. My personal practice is this. I accept lab tests, imaging reports, and all manner of medical records from other states as valid. So why wouldn't I also accept advance directives from other states? When those rare events happen (such as caring for a terminal patient from out of state), I honor the advance directive form regardless of its origin, and that is what I suggest my colleagues do, too.

Consider keeping a digital copy as well. An easy way to do that is to send yourself (and others as appropriate) an email with a copy of your advance directive attached. Doing that will save it in everyone's email in-box for ready access when needed.

Figure 12.1. Carry an advance directive QR code like this one with you.
Courtesy of MyDirectives.com

Figure 12.2. Advance directive QR code on your cell phone.
Courtesy of MyDirectives.com

Occasionally someone is brought to the ER whose identity is unknown, so we have to figure out who this person is and whom to contact. There are protocols for searching wallets, purses, and cell phones to look for relevant information. Without access to this, ER staff must spend time and effort trying to get medical and family contact data, and sometimes that leads to decision-making with incomplete information.

WHEN YOU GET TO THE HOSPITAL

Despite their best intentions, health care providers are not always as well informed as they should be about the legalities of advance directives. It's not so much a problem of resistance as it is one of unfamiliarity. Doctors and nurses are becoming increasingly knowledgeable about this, but there's still a long way to go. That is because advance directives are still relatively uncommon. As an emergency room doctor, I may see only a handful in a year among the hundreds of seriously ill people I treat. If you receive regular care at institutions such as a hospital, nursing home, or hospice, they will want to have a copy. Be sure to send them any updated forms, so they always have your latest version.

You may need to be the one who educates your health care providers about advance directives.

Too often I've seen advance directives not requested or, if obtained, not honored. It can be challenging to explain to an anxious family that it's my responsibility to honor all advance care planning forms, even if the family disagrees.

That's why patients must be their own advocates. Patients should educate themselves about the legal requirements in their state and be sure to have an updated and legally signed form. In fact, you may need to educate your health care providers. As advance directives become more common, providers will become more familiar with them, and following them will become more routine.

Advances in electronic health records ought to make an advance directive as much a part of a medical record as blood pressure readings or a medication list.

An advance directive is only useful when it can be found and applied. Take the important step of making sure all your advance care-planning forms (along with your will) are up to date, available, and accessible to those who will need to have them.

13

Help, We Need Somebody

PROVIDING SUPPORT

———

I think we all have empathy. We may not have
enough courage to display it.
—MAYA ANGELOU

BEING WITH THE SERIOUSLY ILL IS NOT EASY

It's natural to worry about how to be with someone who is seriously ill, but often the most important gift you can bring to these situations is simply your presence. It's astonishing what solace can come to a suffering person from not being alone.

For those in medical settings who are bombarded by tests, procedures, and frequent checking of their vital signs, it is often a joy just to have someone near who is there solely to be with them, with no other agenda (no matter how helpful or necessary those medical agendas are). If you are the visitor, it helps to center yourself and make a conscious effort to let go of any needs or wants of your own and simply keep company with the person.

Counselors, chaplains, and social workers can be valuable resources to help visitors process the stress that these situations can generate. Every medical institution can direct you to these helpers, and there is generally no cost involved.

No matter how strong we think we are, we may need support.

There are many ways to support patients. Animals are experts at living in the moment, and that attitude communicates to humans. I used to bring my own little dog to a nursing home where I was the medical director. A bichon frise, Louie was soft and cuddly, and he seemed to sense what patients needed, whether to pet him or to have him curl up next to them. Sometimes he was the only living being with whom they had affectionate physical contact. Pets on Wheels and similar programs bring well-trained pets to hospitals and nursing homes.

Another service provided by some institutions is therapeutic music. Again, the service is meant to bring pleasure and relaxation to people who are in anxious situations. The greatest gift to many hospital or hospice patients is that of restful sleep, and music can calm the nerves and lead the mind down more peaceful avenues. For those who are near death, a therapeutic musician avoids recognizable melodies and rhythms. Those aspects of music are thought to ground us to life, which is why familiar music is so helpful to those who are in pain and healing. But when someone is dying, that person may desire to let go of life, and it can be moving to see someone appear to float away on the loosely connected notes and chords of a harp or guitar. There is a growing movement by choral societies and single musicians to provide music to the sick and dying.

We can show our support in other ways, such as by bringing a meal, running an errand, or lending an ear to a caregiver who is feeling overwhelmed. There are many websites that facilitate support—from providing home care to organizing the sharing of tasks and schedules. Three examples are Caring Bridge (caring bridge.org), Lots of Helping Hands (lotsofhelpinghands.com), and Take Them a Meal (takethemameal.com).

You're learning what it's like to be human. All humans
are aware of death, so we're all a little bit sad. All the time.
That's just the deal.
—Eleanor Shellstrop in The Good Place

HOW YOU CAN HELP AFTER SOMEONE DIES

Death is such a cataclysmic blow that it can leave us paralyzed, not knowing how to act or even how to feel. When we lose someone close to us, this confusion may be expected. But when someone dies who is at a further remove from us or when the bereavement is not ours but that of a friend or colleague, we may also find ourselves at a loss for how to express our sympathy.

Our culture doesn't prepare us well to deal with other people who are confronting a death. We don't know the "rules of the road." We want to be supportive but not intrusive. We want to be helpful, but we're not sure how to do that. Should we visit in person? Call? Send a note? An email? Flowers? Food? What is our role in the death of a close family member versus a more remote one? What's the right reaction to the death of a family member of a friend or coworker?

The circumstances may dictate different responses. What if the deceased is a baby born with serious birth defects? Or a teenager killed in a car accident? A young victim of an overdose? A middle-aged person who suffers a sudden heart attack? An adult who succumbs after a long battle with cancer? A 90-year-old who dies of old age? These are hard questions with no quick-fix answers, but there are some actions to consider taking.

Attending the funeral or burial ceremony may be appropriate and appreciated by the mourning family. Sending flowers or making a charitable donation in memory of the deceased is a thoughtful way to show sympathy. A note of condolence or a visit to a viewing or to a house of mourning is a more personal way to show concern for those who are grieving, but we may not know what to say when we get there.

There are companies that provide email cards, but to me this feels impersonal. Offering "thoughts and prayers" is genuine, but those stock phrases are getting overused. My approach is to hand-write a short note just to let the bereaved know I'm thinking about them. There's something personal about a handwritten note, a connection that gets lost in our electronic world. Here's a starting point for you to consider: *Please accept my sympathies on the loss of [name]. These are always hard things to deal with, but please know that many friends are thinking of you at this difficult time. If there's anything I can do to help, please let me know.*

For the visitor to a memorial gathering, it's best to take behavioral cues from the mourners.

I usually then add something more personal about the person who died if I knew them well enough, such as a memory of a good time we shared together, a funny situation, or some way in which they affected my life. Such remembrances can be meaningful to the recipient.

Things are a bit different when you are visiting someone in person. For the visitor, it's best to take your cue from the mourners. Allow them to speak and follow their lead. Don't interrupt with stories of your own, even if you think that would be helpful. For example, if someone recently lost a parent, you may be tempted to share how you dealt with that loss, but it's better to offer that only if asked. If they want to talk about their loved one, listen to them or share a story. If they want to talk about something else, join them in that. If they want to be silent, be silent with them. Sometimes, those in mourning don't want to talk at all. In that case, a simple "We are here for you" will suffice. If the mourners have a different religion or spiritual orientation than you do, try to learn a little about those customs before showing up.

Today, social media offer other ways to express sympathy over death. Professor Carla Sofka of Siena College has coined the term "thanatechnology." She writes,

> How society deals with tragedy and loss is being transformed by websites, virtual cemeteries and social media—this is thanatechnology. There are pros and cons to using thanatechnology. For example, the Caring Bridge website provides seriously ill people with a way to quickly share information, provided their family and friends have the link. Messages of support can instantly be posted. Websites and blogs designed to help people cope with tragedy are easy to find, but hopefully the information is trustworthy. Before the digital age, people needing to share "bad news" had control over how and when this was done, often talking with someone face to face or on the telephone. Now, people often learn about a tragedy within minutes via a text message or posting on Facebook or Twitter. Once the news goes public, control over what happens with the information is lost, and some family and friends may learn about the death in a less-than-ideal way. While many people find comfort in sharing memories of the deceased on social media, others who prefer to grieve in private may be forced to deal with powerful reactions in a public place if these postings are unexpected.

We may be unsure about how long after death we should continue to be supportive. In the immediate aftermath there's a rush of attention. Sometimes a bewildering number of people attend a funeral service, overwhelming the bereaved and making it difficult to connect personally. But a few weeks later, the family is alone. This is especially true when a spouse dies, and a few weeks later the surviving spouse is on their own. That might be the best time to show up and provide company, conversation, or an invitation to an activity.

RITUALS AND CUSTOMS

Human cultures everywhere have created rituals of mourning, and these often contain a great deal of psychological wisdom. Some have criticized our contemporary culture for not recognizing a period of mourning or providing a way to let others know that we are in a state of recovering from loss. The death of a close family member can leave a person angry, despairing, anxious, or simply emotionally wrung out, not knowing how to behave or how to feel. Having rules to follow can often be a great comfort.

There are as many ways of managing this process as there are different religions and cultures. Prompt burial is preferred by many cultures, with mourning to follow afterward for a prescribed number of days, weeks, or months. In some cultures, memorial rituals and vigils occur in the days before the funeral and disposition of the body, as with an Irish wake. In others, a service may be held weeks later. These memorial customs, like other traditions, offer a framework for living with our losses.

Most American churches have their own traditions, and their members find comfort in them. They have varying approaches to vigils, wakes, viewings, funerals, and gravesite services. Some of these are specific and detailed. Roman Catholic custom begins the process before the person dies, with the administering of last rites. Interestingly, most religious traditions don't specify how long mourning should last. The Eastern Orthodox traditions are an exception, with prayer rituals prescribed at set dates over time, including an annual memorial service.

Jewish tradition prescribes gradually diminishing levels of mourning. In the day or two after death, the mourner has no obligations other than to arrange for the funeral. After the funeral service, which occurs as quickly as possible, the more formal mourning begins with the 7-day period of "shiva," when friends and family provide food, company, and comfort to the mourners.

Many traditions have ways for the bereaved to indicate their state of mourning, by wearing a black armband or ribbon, for example. Some customs call for hanging a wreath or banner on the front door to indicate the household is in mourning.

But what about those who are not part of any religious or cultural tradition, or who have consciously rejected the tradition they were born into? Over a quarter of the US population now self-designate as "nones": that is, they do not identify with any religion. Some members of this cat-

Rituals are important for the mourners and for the communities we belong to.

egory maintain a belief in a higher power, but the category also includes agnostics and atheists. While religious funeral observances can be comforting to believers, for some people in the none category, attending a religious funeral service can be downright upsetting. For nones it may be even more important to plan any formalities following their own death, as they cannot rely on tradition to do the planning for them.

For many in our secular era, there is a tendency to forgo all ritual, to simply dispose of the body through burial, cremation, or donation, and to hold no service of remembrance. But I would suggest doing otherwise for a couple of reasons.

For one, rituals can give someone the space to accustom themselves gradually to the loss of a loved one. For another, a memorial service or funeral allows others who knew the deceased to remember and to say goodbye in a respectful way.

I experienced this absence of a service myself when my brother Glen died. He had been in ill health, so his death, while heartrending, was not a surprise. He had had no religion, and our mother was so broken up that she didn't want to have anything to do with the arrangements. Although she was religious herself, she emphatically didn't want a memorial service for him, so we didn't have one. But we got calls from Glen's friends and colleagues for weeks afterward. My brother was a musician, and they wanted to talk about him, to play music they had played together, and to be with each other. I think my mother would have gained comfort from the service as well, but that never happened. She remained distraught about Glen for the rest of her life. I learned a lesson from that experience. Rituals are important not only for the mourners but also for the communities of which we are all a part.

PLAN YOUR OWN FUNERAL

Some people pre-plan their funerals down to the last detail. Some plan ahead to the extent of buying cemetery plots or letting loved ones know that they prefer or don't prefer cremation. But many, perhaps the majority of us, avoid planning for the same reasons we avoid completing an advance directive: our fears or superstitions surrounding our own deaths. Yet there can be sound psychological, financial, and spiritual reasons to consider our final passages.

Planning one's own memorial service can be a life-enhancing project. One young woman who was an atheist was so put off by a relative's highly religious funeral that she was moved to begin collecting readings and music that were meaningful to her as a celebration of life, with the thought that they would form the basis of her own memorial service. Some might find this pointless for a young person, but it provided a way for her to consider values and beliefs and to discern what was important.

This raises a question: If you could plan your own funeral, what would you want to happen? For myself, I'd prefer a prompt and simple burial, followed by a memorial service about a month or two later, after the initial grief had faded. At that point, I'd like it to be a recollection with stories of my life, in large part so that my grandchildren would better remember me.

CONTEMPLATION: DEATH AND THE MIRACLE OF LIFE

Many great religious sages have pointed to a contemplation of their own death as the door to profound spiritual insights. For example, the early twentieth-century Hindu teacher Ramana Maharshi told of an experience he had as a teenager:

> I was sitting in a room on the first floor of my uncle's house. I seldom had any sickness and on that day there was nothing wrong with my health, but a sudden, violent fear of death overtook me. There was nothing in my state of health to account for it; and I did not try to account for it or to find out whether there was any reason for the fear. I just felt, "I am going to die," and began thinking what to do about it. It did not occur to me to consult a doctor or my elders or friends. I felt that I had to solve the problem myself, then and there. The shock of the fear of death drove my mind inwards and I said to myself mentally, without actually framing the words: "Now death has come; what does it mean? What is it that is dying? This body dies." And I at once dramatized the occurrence of death. I lay with my limbs stretched out stiff as though rigor mortis had set in and imitated a corpse so as to give greater reality to the enquiry. I held my breath and kept my lips tightly closed so that no sound could escape, so that neither the word "I" nor any other word could be uttered. "Well then," I said to myself, "this body is dead. It will be carried stiff to the burning ground and there burnt and reduced to ashes. But with the death of this body am I dead? Is the body 'I'? It is silent and inert, but I feel the full force of my personality and even the voice of the 'I' within me, apart from it. So I am Spirit transcending the body. The body dies but the Spirit that transcends it cannot be touched by death. This means I am the deathless Spirit." . . . Fear of death had vanished once and for all.

In the Christian tradition, Father Richard Rohr, of the Order of Friars Minor, wrote, "Contemplative prayer is one way to practice imposing silence upon our cares, our desires and our imaginings. Contemplative practice might be five or twenty minutes of 'dying,' of letting go of the small mind in order to experience the big mind, of letting go of the false self in order to experience the True Self, of letting go of the illusion of our separation from God in order to experience our inherent union."

The contemporary new-age teacher Eckhart Tolle wrote of a similar experience of deep contemplation of his own death. It taught him that "Death is a stripping away of all that is not you. The secret of life is to 'die before you die' and find that there is no death."

The people of the Asian nation of Bhutan are known for their Gross National Happiness Index. Akin to our economic measurement of gross national product, the Bhutanese assess government policy by measuring psychological well-being, health, education, good governance, cultural and ecological diversity, living standards, and community vitality. Yet there are also Bhutanese customs suggesting that one think about death five times each day and that the death of a loved one is to be followed by a detailed 49-day mourning period. For the people of Bhutan, the contemplation of death leads to an enhanced appreciation of life.

> That it will never come again is what makes life so sweet.
> —EMILY DICKINSON

14

The Better End

SURVIVING (AND DYING) ON YOUR OWN TERMS IN TODAY'S MODERN MEDICAL WORLD

———

It is as natural to die as to be born.
—FRANCIS BACON

Death twitches my ear; "Live," he says . . . "I'm coming."
—VIRGIL

ABBY MILLER'S STORY: A BETTER END

Abby Miller was 54 years old when she was diagnosed with ovarian cancer, and it hit her hard. A guidance counselor by profession, she had enough presence of mind to know that she needed some support just to hear her primary care doctor's recommendations for care. "I wouldn't have remembered a word," she told her friend Carol. "Once I heard 'cancer,' my brain kind of froze."

Dr. Mitchell had given her referrals to three oncologists and told Abby that choosing one would be an important decision. "After all," he said, "you are going to have a long relationship with this person, so you'll want to be sure you understand each other well. I'll continue to be there for you in any and every way I can, but a specialist is needed now."

Abby was even further distressed. On top of being told about a serious disease, she now had to investigate the world of cancer doctors who accepted her insurance plan. She didn't like the first two she met. She thought one was too cold, and the other seemed too busy to make time to answer all her questions. But Dr. Roberta Reese was just right: pleasant, professional with high ratings, and focused on Abby during their meeting. She was direct and factual with her explanations but also sympathetic.

_____

Find a doctor you can trust and talk to.

_____

Dr. Reese's brother was a cancer survivor, so she understood much of what Abby was going through. She told Abby that each person was different and that making exact predictions was impossible. But at a minimum, Abby could expect several good years ahead.

Abby had been divorced for over 10 years. Her son, Josh, lived 1,500 miles away, where he'd recently started a new job. But she had a large network of friends: some from work, others from her book group or her knitting club; some she'd known ever since high school and college. Carol was the one she was closest to, and it was Carol whom she invited to accompany her to the doctor's office to hear what lay ahead.

The three of them discussed options: surgery, chemotherapy, radiation. Cancer therapy has become increasingly individualized. Cells are studied to determine which modalities or medications will have the best chance of success with a particular type of tumor. This process had already begun in Abby's case. The first step was surgery with a tumor biopsy to analyze the cancer cells, to be followed by chemo. They scheduled the operation for the following week.

Abby wasn't one to hide things. She called Josh in Texas, and she invited her closest friends to a gathering at her home that weekend. Their reactions were shock and dismay, followed by offers of help and support. Abby wasn't sure what kind of help she would need, but she appreciated knowing that they were there for her.

Prior to surgery, Abby obtained an advance directive and began to consider the forms. It felt too soon to be making those decisions, but she decided to name Josh and Carol her joint health care agents. The rest she postponed until after surgery, when she would have a better idea of what she was up against.

Abby underwent a laparotomy, a full opening of the abdomen to get complete access to all internal organs. Her uterus, fallopian tubes, and ovaries were removed. At the same time, her other internal organs were examined, and samples of tissue were obtained to see if the cancer had spread.

Abby spent a few days in the hospital, recuperating from surgery. The biopsy results showed that the cancer had spread but not far. She was a candidate for chemotherapy, but as chemo attacks the most rapidly growing cells, which include those that are repairing wounds, it would have to wait until after her surgical incisions healed. Josh wanted to fly out to be with her, but she assured him she was well taken care of. She told him to wait, to save his vacation and family-leave time for when she might need him more.

Dr. Reese (whom Abby now called Roberta) explained the typical course of her disease. Patients with her type of cancer usually responded well to the first round of chemo and would go into remission. If and when the cancer recurred, as it did in most cases like hers, a second round of chemo would be given. There would most likely be a good response but not one as good as the first round. This cycle would probably repeat two or three more times, but unless she was one of the few lucky ones whose cancer permanently disappeared, there would come a time when nothing more could be done.

Friends pitched in during her surgical recovery and first round of chemo, bringing meals to her at home and helping with errands. Carol used websites that facilitated the sharing of tasks and schedules. Friends rotated in visiting Abby so that she was never alone for long periods, either in her house or during her treatments at the cancer clinic. Her job allowed flexible leave time, so Abby was able to continue helping the students she counseled. She joined a local support group of cancer patients, where she met other people in the same circumstances. Sharing emotions and life stories brought her comfort.

The days after chemo were particularly hard. Abby was not so vain as to mind the resultant hair loss. She was amused that people thought she looked better in her new wig than she had with her own hair. But the nausea and fatigue were tough, and she struggled through those long days and nights.

Josh wanted her to get "everything possible" in terms of treatment, including any experimental or research protocols. He argued, "at least you will be helping someone else, if not yourself." That sounded good in theory, but when Abby was at the low point in her chemo cycle, the idea of going through horrible symptoms on the off chance it would help someone else in the future felt unreasonable.

Abby returned to her advance directive. She struggled with the part about how much care to receive. She wanted every chance at survival, but she didn't want to suffer if there was no hope of recovery. At this point she certainly would want CPR if she experienced a cardiac or respiratory emergency. She finally decided that she would continue with treatment only as long as she could hope to live with meaningful functioning and a reasonable quality of life. But what did "a reasonable quality of life" mean for Abby?

Abby came to the conclusion that there were three things she especially loved that, for her, might define quality of life. The first was her dog, Mick, a scruffy poodle-terrier mix. Taking him for walks in the morning and evening was a highlight of her day, as was brushing his coat and cuddling with him in bed in the morning. Her second love was music. Abby liked all kinds of music, from opera to rock, and she could spend hours listening to music, going from one genre to another. The third was chocolate. Abby's favorite indulgence was two squares of dark chocolate after dinner. Along with the company of her loved ones, these daily rituals buoyed her mood through her illness. If she could no longer enjoy them, she would know that she was beyond a reasonable quality of life.

As the months progressed, Abby settled into the reality of living with cancer. Despite all the pain, nausea, and anxiety, Abby eventually began to see herself as blessed in a peculiar way. She was no longer a victim; she was a survivor. Her appreciation for life was enhanced, and she savored every moment. Going to the movies with friends became a joyful experience, more than just a night out. She had always been good at her counseling job, but her own struggles seemed to give her more empathy for her students and their problems. Things that had troubled her before became minor inconveniences, or even occasions for laughter. One day Abby was in line at a supermarket checkout counter. The line was moving slowly because the person in front of her was trying to decide between two items and then fumbling to find a credit card. In the past, Abby would have thought, "What an idiot. They had all this time in the store to make a choice and then stood in line for 5 minutes without thinking to check for the credit card." Abby would have been fuming. But now, she took it in stride. She had found a new capacity for patience.

What would define "quality of life" for you?

Most precious of all, her relationship with her son deepened. They were able to speak of their love for each other in a way that hadn't been possible before. And Josh was able to talk more openly to his mother about his own life. Two years into her battle with cancer, Abby traveled cross-country for Josh's wedding to his girlfriend, Emma. She shed bittersweet tears, grateful to be present at his marriage but thinking of what she might not live to see.

This went on for 4 and a half years, through three rounds of chemo. In between, Abby returned to normal life. Then Abby began to notice differences. Her pain was not responding as well to the pain medications. Her clothes hung on her thinning frame as she lost more weight. Breathing was getting harder, and she tired more quickly. Her walks with Mick the dog got shorter and less frequent. Eventually she hired a dog walker to take over.

One day she woke up with abdominal discomfort. This had happened before, but now it was worse. As the day progressed, she knew something was really wrong. Her belly bloated out, and the crampy pain increased. At 3 p.m., Carol took her to the emergency room. The diagnosis was a blocked bowel, a known complication of ovarian cancer and its treatment. Plus, she had become dehydrated, and her body chemistries were out of line. A tube was put down her nose into her stomach, removing air and fluid, and that eased the pressure and bloating. She was admitted to the intensive care unit.

Sometimes a tube will clear the problem, but after the initial relief, her condition was not improving. After 2 days, it was clear that surgery was required. Without it, death was certain to come from the infection the bowel blockage would cause. The surgeon was confident that Abby would survive the operation. Disoriented by the pain medications she'd been given, Abby struggled to understand what was going on. She could hardly imagine another operation. The first one had been tough enough, but she had been in pretty good shape back then. What would happen this time, when she was already in a weakened condition? She began to cry.

Who would decide what to do? At least one doctor was concerned that Abby was incompetent to make this decision, given her pain and heavy medication. Josh had flown in, and he and Carol considered the options. Was this a lifesaving procedure or an effort at futile heroics? They agreed to go forward with the operation, and it was successful.

Abby awoke in the surgical recovery room. She was disoriented and groggy. The next few days were a fog, but she made a slow recovery. Eventually she was able to go home, but she resolved never to go through that again.

Four months after the surgery, the oncologist told her that the cancer was spreading again and that the only possibility for stopping it lay with an untried experimental drug. Abby knew that she had reached the end. There was no timetable, but the doctor told her that death would most likely be soon.

Abby asked how the end might come. Dr. Reese told her she might die from kidney or liver failure, as both organs were riddled with metastatic cancer. Or a growing tumor might erode into a large blood vessel, causing internal bleeding. Or she could develop an infection, probably pneumonia, as the final cause of death.

The financial paperwork had been completed, but Abby still had two issues to settle. The first was to update her advance directive to reflect that she no longer wanted 911 called in case of an emergency, nor did she want CPR. The second issue was a related one: where to die. Abby had spoken with others who had lost loved ones to cancer, and she had thought long and hard about what she wanted for herself.

ABBY'S DECISIONS

She spoke with Josh and Carol about her decisions. She told them she was no longer a candidate for treatment. She didn't want to undergo any more surgery or chemo. She only wanted pain medicines, personal care, and comfort.

At first Josh was upset with her decision. Why refuse CPR? What about that experimental treatment? Why give up early? He and Emma were planning to have a child in the near future. Didn't Abby want to keep fighting to live long enough to see her first grandchild?

"Of course, I want to know your children," Abby told him. "But this is not within my control. Or yours either." She brought out a folder and handed it to him. "I knew that you and Emma would have children one day and that I probably wouldn't be around to see them grow up. Carol and I made a video. In here is a DVD with a message for my grandchildren: things I want them to know but won't be there to share with them in person."

Through his tears, Josh nodded his acceptance. He could see how his mother was suffering. As sad as it was for him, in good conscience he couldn't ask her to prolong the ordeal.

Returning to her advance directive, Abby read what she had written: "I only want food and pain medicine, and if I get too weak to eat, I don't want artificial feeding. I want to be kept clean and comfortable, and I prefer that this care come as much as possible from those closest to me. I want to die at home, not in a hospital. I ask that my favorite music be present in my last days and that Mick be allowed to be with me as long as possible. If my heart should stop beating or I stop breathing, stay with me and allow me to die in peace. I don't want you to ever feel guilty. By following my instructions, you are showing your love for me."

An advance directive form can guide you, but you can add to it as much as you want to make your wishes clear.

Abby didn't want to die in an institution, no matter how homelike it tried to be. She hadn't come to these decisions lightly. Early on in Abby's illness, Dr. Reese had suggested that she meet with a nurse from the hospital's supportive care program. They had helped Abby deal with the discomforts that came with chemo and radiation therapy. They had also given her information about hospice programs available both in institutions and at home. Abby began working with hospice and had found that the nurses and other staff members helped greatly in every aspect of her care. She appreciated their attention and professionalism. The care she got at home was excellent. She was also fortunate that Josh could take family leave, and Carol and other friends took turns in staying with her.

As her last weeks approached, Abby talked with Josh and Carol about the kind of funeral she wanted. She didn't believe in spending money on an expensive casket or on embalming. Her faith that her spirit would live on after death had become stronger over the course of her illness, but she wanted her physical remains to be returned to the earth as quickly and naturally as possible.

ABBY'S WAY

Josh had been impressed by the wake held at home for Emma's uncle the previous year. It was comforting for Emma to pay her respects in the house where her uncle had lived, instead of in a funeral parlor. Older relatives had commented that wakes always used to be held at home.

Abby said that she would prefer a home wake, too, if Carol and her other friends were willing to do that for her. She liked the idea of her body being cared for at the end by the hands of those who loved her. Carol talked to the circle of Abby's friends, who agreed that they would be honored to perform this last service for Abby. Abby left it to Josh and Carol to plan the funeral service, asking only that some of her favorite pieces of music be played. The burial would take place in the newly opened natural burial section of a local cemetery, with a simple engraved river stone to mark her grave.

It was early November, but Abby decided to decorate for the holidays. She had always loved doing that, and she didn't know whether she'd make it to late December. Her cancer had taught her to appreciate life during every moment, to give and receive happiness at every opportunity. She wanted her last weeks to be brightened by lights and greenery and the ornaments collected and cherished over a lifetime.

During the next weeks Abby became too weak to leave her house, then too weak to leave her bedroom, and finally too weak to leave her bed. The hospice staff showed Josh, Carol, and the other helpers how to attend to Abby's hygiene needs, how to make the bed with her in it, and how to change her clothes easily.

With Mick nestled at her feet, Abby grew quiet and contemplative, listening to her favorite music, reading when she had the strength. She reflected on all the joys of her life and the people she had known. Sometimes she could almost feel the presence in the room of her own mother and father, who had died years before.

Friends and colleagues came to visit. Some would bring a special chocolate bar for her, and she would take a tiny bite, savoring the rich flavor. Frequently, this candy was the only thing she ate all day. Sometimes the visitors would just sit with her in silence, but often Abby took the opportunity to bestow a small gift from her pottery collection, a piece of advice, and always a loving farewell.

One friend arranged for visits by a volunteer harpist who provided music for the very sick. The lilting tones of old melodies comforted Abby and everyone with her at the house.

As the days went by, her breathing became raspy. The hospice staff adjusted the dose of narcotics so that Abby was comfortable and pain free without being overly sedated. Eventually she began to lapse in and out of consciousness, and the periods of sleep grew longer. She was calm and at peace. Then, late one afternoon as the sun was setting, she slipped under the waves. With Josh holding her hand, she died, surrounded by loving friends.

After Abby had breathed her last, the hospice nurse bathed and dressed her body. Carol and the others laid Abby out in her bed and prepared to welcome the friends who would stop by to pay their respects. Two days later, the family and friends helped lay Abby in her casket and transported her to the chapel for the funeral service and burial.

The end was still difficult for those left behind, but even as they grieved, they found comfort in the time they'd spent with Abby through the dying process. It made the loss more bearable.

Her passing had been a deeply moving experience that would stay with them for as long as they lived.

During the long drive with Mick back to their Dallas home, Josh and Emma talked about how much they'd appreciated Abby's attitude: her openness about her situation, her refusal to collapse into depression, and her joy in life no matter what was happening. She had given them the gift of seeing death as a meaningful part of the arc of a full life.

The best of both worlds: taking full advantage of modern medical science and going out on your own terms when the time comes.

Abby achieved the better end, the best of both worlds. She took full advantage of modern medical science. She found a physician who was competent and compassionate. She allowed others to help her as necessary. She did not treat her disease as something to be ashamed of, but on the other hand, she did not allow it to define her existence. She did not let it stop her from living and enjoying the good things around her. As a result, she survived longer than expected, and her positive attitude played a key role. When the end was in sight, she went out on her own terms. By doing so, she also provided a deeply meaningful life experience for those around her. If there is such a thing, hers was a good death. With planning, more of us can have this experience.

15

Speaking Personally

—

Just as when we come into the world, when we die we are afraid of the unknown. But the fear is something from within us that has nothing to do with reality. Dying is like being born: just a change.
—Isabel Allende, The House of the Spirits

MY NEAR-DEATH EXPERIENCE

As a kid growing up, I remember starting to think about death at about age 12 or 13. No matter how hard I tried to think about death and what happened after, I kept running into an impenetrable wall, and so I gave up the process. But like most kids, I thought of myself as pretty indestructible. Death was something that wouldn't happen to me for a very long time, if ever. So why think about it now?

Over the years, I've worked at maintaining a healthy weight, and my cholesterol levels were good. Since my twenties I have been a sometimes serious runner. To celebrate turning 50, I completed two marathons. A diagnostic cardiac catheterization showed my coronary arteries to be in good shape.

My inner health dialogue was that I was invincible, cardio-vascular-wise. I could run long distances, control my weight, and was doing just fine. That led to creeping overconfidence about what good shape I was in and a belief that I was protected from any possible heart condition. But little by little, over the years, my weight crept up, and my exercise frequency drifted downward.

Early on Saturday morning, March 19, 2016, I was getting dressed at our rental home in Annapolis, Maryland, where we spent most days during the legislative session. Quite suddenly, I felt a hot painful burning in my chest. I began to sweat, and this was not just a sweat of anxiety.

Don't hesitate to call 911 if you are having severe symptoms. I did, and it saved my life.

My shirt was drenched as I began to drip from every pore. I knew something bad was happening, so I called to Shelley to come upstairs. "I'm having chest pain," I told her. "You need to drive me to the hospital." But almost as soon as I'd spoken, I recognized that the situation required more urgent action. "No, forget that. Call 911." It was something I'd preached to patients for years. When in doubt, get to the hospital as fast as you can. If it turns out to be nothing, you might feel a little embarrassed, but pain or numbness can all too often be the first sign of a heart attack or stroke. Seconds count in these situations, and false alarms are a cheap price to pay for ensuring that treatment is prompt. Fortunately, the local ambulance company was nearby, and within a few minutes they had arrived at our house.

Despite the pain, I made it downstairs, and the paramedics put me on a gurney and into the back of the vehicle. They hooked up a monitor and started an IV. Shelley got in the front passenger seat, and off we went.

The paramedics did an EKG to check the electrical activity of my heart. I asked to see it, and it was bad. The tracing showed ST elevations, signs of an acute anterior myocardial infarction. A heart attack, a big one, in the most vulnerable part of the heart. That particular set of tracings is sometimes called "tombstoning" for its characteristic curves that look like grave markers. Shelley was watching me. I looked up at her and made a casual thumbs-down gesture. I even was able to grin. She didn't grin back. Although I knew I was in serious trouble, I felt no panic. It was a strange, somewhat detached feeling.

The paramedics sent the EKG ahead to Anne Arundel Medical Center, as we sped up Main Street to the hospital. On any other day or time, the narrow street would be crowded with cars and pedestrians, but as it was early Saturday morning, there was no traffic. We arrived at the emergency room, and as I was pushed through the facility, my ER physician self, by longtime habit, couldn't help but take note of how the ER was set up. Fortunately it was not at all busy, and I was quickly taken back to a room filled with nurses and staff.

It so happened that the cardiologist on call for emergency cases was in the hospital that morning doing some paperwork. He'd been paged and arrived about a minute after I did. Dr. Jonathan Altschuler took one look at me and the EKG and said, "Let's get this guy up to the cath lab." The "cath lab" is the cardiac catheterization operative suite, where in-depth evaluations of heart function are assessed and treated. Catheters are long thin tubes that are threaded into the heart. Dye is injected and X-ray pictures taken. This shows the anatomy of the heart and its vessels.

While the nurses were getting me ready to be transferred upstairs, Dr. Altschuler went to speak with Shelley: "Your husband is having a very bad heart attack." It was true, and it was also a way to prepare her for the worst-case scenario.

Shelley came into the prep room to be with me. As they hooked me up to monitors and started a second IV, I remembered that I had been named "Legislator of the Year" by the Maryland Nurses Association, and I thought this would be a good thing to share so that the staff would be extra nice to me. And ridiculous as it sounds, I did. The nurses chuckled as they continued with their preparations. I imagine they were thinking, "This guy is dying, and he's telling us about his awards." In the same unreal vein, I asked

Shelley to let certain legislators know that I wouldn't be in that day. I was responsible for several issues that would be debated on the House floor, and I wanted someone else to get the files and be prepared. Again, ridiculous. There I was, having a heart attack and worrying about some legislation.

I was wheeled into an elevator, then down the hall to the cath lab, where I slid off the gurney onto the operating table. Dr. Altschuler wasn't waiting for anything. He started preparing my right groin (femoral artery and vein) for a catheter insertion; there was no time to waste.

The next thing I remember was waking up in a hospital bed. My groin was sore, and I felt a bit goofy, but everything was all right. No pain, no symptoms. Apparently, the procedure went swiftly and well. A plaque inside my left main coronary artery had ruptured and blocked the blood flow. Another term for this particular event is "widow maker," which indicates the usual outcome. The doctor removed the obstruction and placed a stent, thus restoring flow in the artery, and my EKG returned to normal. There were no other blockages. It was now 9:30 a.m., barely 2 hours after my first symptoms.

I spent 2 days in the hospital being monitored. My cardiac enzymes (chemicals in the blood that measure heart damage) rose a little. Other tests showed no damage. As explained to me, it was like being "kicked in the heart." There was a bruise, and it would heal. On Wednesday, I returned to work.

I reflected on how many things had to go right for me, one after another, to have escaped death with essentially no consequences. It was a Saturday morning. I had the good sense to ask for a 911 call without delay. The fire station was close by and not busy. The paramedics arrived within minutes and had the best equipment, training, and skills. There was no traffic to delay us in getting to the hospital, and all the key personnel were in the ER upon my arrival. The procedure went smoothly. If any single one of these things had been different, I'd either be dead or living with a damaged heart. If I had been at our home in Baltimore, travel time from fire station to home to hospital would have been 40 minutes at minimum, instead of less than 15. At another time or day, there could have been delays in a busy ER. Traffic could have slowed us down. The cardiologist could have been out or tied up in another procedure. As it happened for me, there was no waiting for the cardiologist, and he acted swiftly and surely. Another medical maxim about heart attacks: "time is muscle," meaning that delays in care can have negative consequences. My wife, Shelley, put it another way: "All your guardian angels were on duty that morning."

In retrospect, what astonished me was that at no point did I feel anxious or panicky. Both would have been appropriate reactions, but I didn't have them. I just felt that I was present and that whatever was going to happen would happen, and there was nothing I could do about it. (If only I could generate that same emotion for other life trials.) Is there something about death being close that triggers a biochemical reaction? Could something be programmed in our DNA that kicks in when death is near? Had my brain been flooded with calming endorphins? There is some evidence that humans and animals alike are flooded with endorphins after a serious injury. Some have speculated that perhaps this facilitates the taking of protective action for either the self or for family members in an emergency.

I'd seen this sort of calm reaction once when watching a deer die in the forest. Mortally wounded, it just bleated softly, rolled over, and breathed its last. I'd also seen people die, and many times I noted how calm they were.

WHAT I LEARNED AND WHAT I'D CHOOSE FOR MYSELF

To say this event was a wake-up call would be an understatement. I changed my eating habits, reignited my exercise regimen with regular running and swimming, added yoga and meditation to my weekly schedule, started a weight-lifting program guided by a trainer at my local gym, and lost 40 lbs. While none of us can avoid dying, we can make our lives healthier and more comfortable.

Months later, I began to reflect. Was I saved for some reason? How do I make meaning of this, or was it just dumb luck? And when other people die, do they experience the calm letting-go feeling I had, or do they experience something else? Does that only apply to medical conditions? What if I were in a plummeting plane about to crash? I think I'd be panicking then, but who knows?

To say this event was a wake-up call would be an understatement.

I'd like to believe that there is something that helps us over the transition, no matter the particular circumstances. Perhaps someday scientists will identify the specific chemical or neural pathway that does this. As nature seems to have designed us for life, it would seem logical that it would also provide for us in death.

People often ask about my personal views on death and dying. What are my values when it comes to end-of-life choices? What would I take into account, or what would I want my health care agent to take into account, if such decisions needed to be made?

The first questions for me—as for many people—would be these: Is my mind working? Do I have consciousness, even if somewhat impaired? Second, I'd ask, what's going on with my body? Am I in pain? How much care do I need? Have I become a burden to my loved ones? Am I so debilitated that every bodily function requires support? And third, what is the context of my life? Am I surrounded by family and friends? Or am I living in an isolated situation in an institution?

I don't mind pondering these questions or providing my answers. If I can't demonstrate a willingness to being open and honest about these issues, I can't ask others to do the same.

If my mind were functional and my pain tolerable, then I would want to be kept alive as long as possible, using every modality reasonably available. I've also specified other items that are important to me. For example, my advance directive says that I want to be taken outside frequently or at least have a view of nature if possible. I want to have full control of the TV remote. I have an electronic picture display that cycles through hundreds of family photos, which I enjoy watching for a few minutes each day, even now while I'm in good health. I find it soothing and cheering, so I'd want that at my bedside. I'd want family and friends around as much as possible. But, if I can only look forward to bare survival, without mental capacity or a reasonable hope of regaining functions, or if I'm in extreme pain, then I would want only those measures taken that would keep me comfortable. In such a case I would not want artificial nutrition to prolong my life. At that point, if I developed a serious illness, I'd let nature take its course.

Most health providers I know who work in emergency or critical-care medicine have completed an advance directive. Why? Because we've seen what happens when people don't. While we've seen amazing cures and recoveries, we've also seen the people who get something called "care," when it's really closer to torture. Medicine is a science that requires human judgment. There comes a time when enough is enough, when we cross over the line separating meaningful care from the humility to let nature take over.

THIS IS SO IMPORTANT FOR OURSELVES AND OUR FAMILIES

I urge everyone over the age of 18 to complete an advance directive. The websites in the Resources section will help you find the form you need. Take the time to think about what care you would want, consult with people whose advice you respect, and then complete the form and make it legally valid. Be sure to let other people know where your advance directive is kept. Give a copy to your doctor and to your health care agent. And, should your wishes or circumstances change, update your advance directive as often as you like.

It costs nothing. Completing, legalizing, and distributing these forms is free or of minimal cost and takes only a few minutes, but the benefits are invaluable.

I have made many presentations on a variety of medical issues, including a health policy series at the Johns Hopkins Bloomberg School of Public Health. This series covers a range of health care policy topics. Most of the people in attendance are graduate students at the school, who compose a diverse group of brilliant men and women from this country and abroad, generally in their twenties or thirties. Many already have a graduate degree in another field. They are doctors, nurses, lawyers, social workers, scientists, or people who work in business or public policy fields. This combination of accomplished professionals leads to some interesting discussions about ethics, economics, and politics, as well as medical science.

When we cover end-of-life care, I ask how many of them have completed an advance directive. Usually just a few hands go up, never more than 20% of the audience. I then ask them to find a suitable form and go through the process of completing it. I think it's important to have a personal experience of doing something, when possible, if you are going to discuss it with others and take a position on their decisions. If you are serious about a career in health care, I firmly believe that you have to be consistent, lead by example, and do those things personally that you advise others to do.

Completing an advance directive connects a person more closely to life and death. The process helps us recognize our basic values. My students have thanked me for prodding them into doing it. Many have told me that completing an advance directive changed their view of the health care system and the people in it. They developed a better rapport with patients and health care providers, and an appreciation of the difficult choices involved.

One said, "I now have a greater sense of empathy for every human being." Some decided to be the change agent and bring the topic up to their own families.

I kept a stack of advance directive forms in my legislative office. I'd ask everyone who came to lobby me about a health care issue if they had completed one. If they had not, I'd suggest that it was one essential step only they could take. No one could do that for them. To me, this is a key personal part of being an advocate. Passionate advocates ought to model responsible behavior because it increases their credibility and effectiveness when they do.

In the closing comments of my presentations, I ask members of the audience whether they will now complete their own forms if they haven't done so already, and almost all agree to do it. Then I tell them that they are now deputized to be the ones to bring this up to others. That personal connection can be quite persuasive.

I wrote this book with my wife because we believe that everyone needs to learn how to survive, and eventually to die, in today's modern medical world.

The consequences of our decisions can be far reaching. Will our loved ones spend years at our bedside agonizing over decisions? Will arduous and painful—but ultimately futile—treatment be administered because no one was there to direct our care? Will end-of-life expenses bankrupt our family? Will family conflicts erupt because we did not take the time to express our wishes when we were able to do so?

It doesn't have to be this way. The actions we take to make known our wishes for our end-of-life care greatly affect the happiness, well-being, and finances of those nearest to us. Death is universal, but families are better off when they live through a deliberately and thoughtfully planned process of a loved one's passage from life to death. Not only are they often able to bond with each other in the face of their grief, but also, years later, they may look back with reverence on the experience.

I believe that, as a culture, we are in denial of death. We desperately need to enhance our empathy with our fellow beings as they make this transition. Too many of us don't know how to respond or are uncomfortable in responding to a friend or family member in the throes of dying. We have trouble showing our support to those in mourning for a recent loss. By emerging from our cultural denial of death, we open ourselves to greater empathy, helpfulness, and appreciation of life. As psychotherapist Josefine Speyer has noted, "When we embrace death as a part of life, we also embrace the ill, the dying, and the bereaved as partners in living."

We have been given a gift: the opportunity to participate actively in the drama of life's final passage.

We need to seize the best of both worlds: the best that medical care has to offer combined with the personal experience of life's natural end. We should strive for life and health for everyone with all the tools that science and ingenuity and compassion can offer. Then, when the end is approaching—as it does for all of us—we should use that same science, ingenuity, and compassion to bring comfort and dignity to the dying and their survivors.

We have been given a gift: the opportunity to actively participate in the drama of life's final passage. To prepare for it, we need to take action by carefully considering and completing an advance directive and then sharing those values with others (figure 15.1).

Figure 15.1. Example of an advance directive form

There are many versions of advance directives, but they all have these basic components in common.

FIRST: The kind of care I want if I can't make those decisions for myself

If I have a terminal condition:

Life-sustaining treatments

_____ I do not want life-sustaining treatments (including CPR) started. If these have been started, then stop them.

_____ I want life-sustaining treatments to the fullest extent possible.

_____ Let my doctors decide what's best for me.

_____ Allow natural death.

Artificial nutrition and hydration

_____ I do not want artificial nutrition and hydration started if these would be the main treatments keeping me alive. If these have been started, then stop them.

_____ I want artificial nutrition and hydration even if they are the main treatments keeping me alive.

Comfort care

_____ I want to be kept as comfortable and free of pain as possible, even if such care prolongs my dying or shortens my life.

_____ Provide pain and anxiety medicines, including medical cannabis if allowed in this state, as needed to keep me comfortable.

If I am in a persistent vegetative state with no hope of recovery:

Life-sustaining treatments

_____ I do not want life-sustaining treatments (including CPR) started. If these have been started, then stop them.

_____ I want life-sustaining treatments.

_____ Let my doctors decide what's best for me.

Figure 15.1 (*cont.*)

Artificial nutrition and hydration

_____ I do not want artificial nutrition and hydration started if they would be the main treatments keeping me alive. If these have been started, then stop them.

_____ I want artificial nutrition and hydration even if these are the main treatments keeping me alive.

Comfort care

_____ I want to be kept as comfortable and free of pain as possible, even if such care prolongs my dying or shortens my life.

Additional directions for any of the above: _____

For all of the above, consult with my health care agent(s).

SECOND: These are my health care agents

My primary health care agent is _____

If the person above cannot or will not make decisions for me, then my secondary health care agent is _____

Other people I designate as health care agents, in order, are _____

I direct that my health care team provide all medical information to my health care agents;

OR, I direct that my health care team provide all medical information to my health care agents, except the following: _____

I request that my health care agent consult with the following people before making medical decisions on my behalf: _____

Other directions

Here are further instructions about my health care: _____

continued

Figure 15.1 (*cont.*)

THIRD: Other choices

A. Organ donation

_____ I do not wish to donate any of my organs or tissues.

_____ I want to donate all of my organs and tissues.

_____ I want to donate only these organs and tissues: _____

Other wishes: _____

B. Autopsy

_____ I do not want an autopsy.

_____ I agree to an autopsy if my doctors recommend it.

_____ I agree to an autopsy if my health care agent deems it useful.

Other wishes: _____

C. Other statements about my medical care

Here are other things I want respected as I approach the end of life:

_____

FOURTH: Making it legal with signatures

Requirements differ from state to state, so check with yours. Generally, you and two witnesses must sign this document to make it legal. Some states require notarization.

A. Your signature

I confirm with my signature that I understand this advance directive document and that it accurately reflects my wishes in accordance with state and federal law.

Signature: _____

Date: _____

Address: _____

Figure 15.1 (*cont.*)

B. Witnesses' signatures

The person who signed this document did so in my presence or sent it to me electronically, consistent with state law. I believe this person to be emotionally and mentally competent to execute this advance directive. I am not related and am not connected financially to this person.

Witness #1

Signature: _____

Date: _____

Address: _____

Witness #2

Signature: _____

Date: _____

Address: _____

An advance directive can be changed at any time. The most recent properly completed version is the one that is in force. Make your advance directive easily available to those who need to know what it says: your doctors (and other health care providers) and your health care agent(s).

Acknowledgments

Whether taking care of patients in a hospital emergency room or shepherding a bill through the legislative process, both are cooperative efforts, impossible to achieve by oneself. The same is true of a book. This one has been a joint effort of me and my wife, Shelley. We worked together on every phase of this project, as we did for my previous book, *The Better End: Surviving (and Dying) on Your Own Terms in Today's Modern Medical World*.

As a physician, I'm thankful to all the patients who entrusted me with their care. It's a privilege to be able to help people dealing with everything from the most minor conditions to life-threatening illness and injury. They have taught me much.

As a Maryland state legislator for 24 years, I am appreciative of the citizens of Maryland's Eleventh District who gave me their trust, their advice, and their votes. It's impossible for any legislator to be an expert on all issues, and input from constituents is always helpful. The public may not realize how much legislators depend on hearing from them.

Shelley and I were helped in creating my previous book by the late Dr. Maya Angelou, who honored us with her wisdom, inspiration, and friendship.

This book began with a research project that evolved from my work at the Johns Hopkins Bloomberg School of Public Health. I was ably assisted by Keshia Pollack Porter, Clarence Lam, Shannon Frattaroli, Michael Klag, David Fakunle, and Ellen MacKenzie.

Many medical colleagues provided wisdom and support, especially Michael Auerbach, who gave freely of his time and experience.

Others who helped include Penny McDougal, Jodi Luby, Anne Evans, Cathy Hamel, Reggie Bodner, Karen Kennedy, Charlie Alexander, Chanee Fabius, Nellie Burke, Robert Donegan, Steve Salamon, Miriam MacGillis, Lorinda Belzberg, Tricia Christensen, Michelle Bernstein, Anne Marie Gustafson, Debbie Miran, Neill

Franklin, Mary Lynn McPherson, Jason Poling, Paula Singer, Laurie Christman, Michael Merson, Marc Katlic, Jeff Zucker, Ben Pomerantz, Bonnie Pastor, and Edo Banach.

Thanks also to Johns Hopkins University Press, especially Joe Rusko and Jackie Wehmueller, without whom none of this would be possible.

We were supported throughout by our family, especially our daughters, Emily, Sarah, and Lizz Morhaim, as well as our son-in-law Ryan Samul and Nancy and Henry Abrams. We miss our beloved brother Steve and sister Mary Lou Cole, who taught us so much in life and death.

Glossary

advance directive: A free legal form completed by an adult person at any age that outlines their choices for medical care should they become unable to make their own decisions.

Affordable Care Act (ACA): A federal legislative overhaul of the US health care system, passed in 2010, that increased the number of Americans covered by health insurance and that, among other reforms, protected those with preexisting conditions; informally known as Obamacare.

Alzheimer's disease: The most common and well-known form of dementia.

amyotrophic lateral sclerosis (ALS): A progressive disease of no known cause in which nerves that stimulate muscles deteriorate, leading to paralysis; also known as Lou Gehrig's disease.

AND (allow natural death): An instruction for medical personnel to let a patient's illness take its natural course, likely leading to death.

angina: Chest pain caused by a lack of blood flow to the heart, which can be a warning sign of a heart attack.

arrhythmia: Irregular beating of the heart, of which there are many types.

artificial nutrition and hydration: Food and water given to a person via a tube inserted through the nose and down into the stomach (NG-tube) or a tube implanted directly into the stomach (G-tube).

assisted dying: A legal right in some states and countries whereby a person, in specific circumstances, ends their own life.

assisted suicide: A death in which someone has helped the deceased take their own life.

autopsy: A dissection and examination of a deceased body and its tissues to determine the cause of death.

BiPAP (bilevel positive airway pressure): A machine that helps push air into the lungs.

CAKE: A website that provides advance directive forms.

cannabis: The marijuana plant or its chemical derivatives used as a medication to relieve a variety of symptoms.

cardiac care unit (CCU): An area in a hospital where patients with serious heart disease get care.

cardiopulmonary resuscitation (CPR): A series of intense medical procedures designed to save a person from dying from failed breathing, a stopped heart, or both.

CAT (computerized axial tomography) scan: An X-ray test that uses a computer to generate complete cross-sectional images of any body part; also referred to as a CT scan.

catheter: Typically a thin, flexible plastic tube inserted into a body part, such as a blood vessel or the urinary tract, to provide an artificial conduit.

code status: Predetermination of whether someone will get a full resuscitation effort, partial intervention, or nothing at all should that person go into cardiac or respiratory arrest.

comfort care: Keeping a person as comfortable as possible without attempting to cure the underlying illness; generally this includes measures such as moistening the person's lips and mouth and administering pain-relieving medicines.

death panel: A popular term, with no basis in reality, in the public discourse about health care reform in 2009, which imagined that a committee, formed by government and empowered by law, would determine when to terminate patient care.

dementia: A condition, of many possible causes, in which the brain's functions of memory, thinking, and self-awareness gradually fail.

DNA (deoxyribonucleic acid): The chemical in organisms that governs the division, differentiation, and function of cells and that carries all genetic information.

DNR (do not resuscitate): A medical order not to perform medical procedures intended to restart a patient's breathing or a stopped heart, an order equivalent to "no CPR."

Donate Life America: A national organization that provides information about and promotes organ donation.

durable power of attorney for health care: Legal authorization for someone to make medical decisions for another person in the event that person becomes unable to make their own decisions.

embalming: A method of preserving a body after death in which all blood and fluids are drained from the circulatory system and replaced with formaldehyde and other chemicals.

emergency room (ER): An area in a hospital where any person can go with any problem at any time; sometimes called an emergency department.

Five Wishes: A source for advance directive documents and information.

full code: A status, by choice or by default, in which someone receives full cardiopulmonary resuscitation if their heart stops beating or they cease to breathe.

health care agent: A person designated by someone to make medical decisions for them in the event they are unable to make those decisions for themselves.

hospice: Care services provided for those with a terminal condition in the last 6 months of their life, typically paid for by Medicare and provided at a facility or at home.

intensive care unit (ICU): An area in a hospital where the sickest patients receive care.

intubation: Insertion of a plastic tube through the mouth and into the trachea (windpipe) to support breathing.

leukemia: A cancer of white blood cells.

living will: Another term for an advance directive.

Medicaid: A government health plan, sponsored by the US federal government and the states, that covers health care for people with limited income and children without other coverage.

Medical Orders for Life-Sustaining Treatment (MOLST): A medical care plan available in some US states for someone with an advanced illness at any stage that is signed by a licensed medical professional (not necessarily a doctor); compare POLST.

Medicare: A US federal government health insurance plan for those who are 65 years of age or older and for some with serious disabling diseases.

MRI (magnetic resonance imaging): An imaging technique that uses magnetic fields and radio waves to generate complete cross-sectional views of any body part.

MyDirectives.com: A website that provides advance directive forms.

narcotic: A drug that reduces awareness and induces sleep, typically an opioid but may be another chemical compound with the same effect.

National Healthcare Decisions Day: A nationally recognized day, April 16 every year, intended to increase public awareness of the options in end-of-life care decisions.

natural burial: Burying a body in a simple and environmentally sensitive manner.

nitroglycerin: A long-used medicine for treating angina chest pain, typically taken under the tongue, which helps to open up the vessels supplying blood to heart muscle.

no CPR: A medical order not to provide cardiopulmonary resuscitation.

nonsteroidal anti-inflammatory drug (NSAID): A medicine, such as ibuprofen, that relieves pain, fever, and inflammation; most drugs of this kind are available without a prescription.

notary public: A person authorized to authenticate signatures on legally binding documents.

opioid: Also known as an opiate, this class of medicines, originally derived from the opium poppy, effectively relieves pain but carries risks of side effects, overdose, and addiction.

organ and tissue donation: Taking organs or tissues from one person and transplanting them in another person to replace what is damaged or dysfunctional.

pacemaker: An electronic device, typically implanted in the chest wall, that sustains heartbeat by transmitting electrical impulses over wires.

palliative care: Care designed to relieve symptoms of pain and stress at any stage of recovery from illness or injury, ideally delivered by a multidisciplinary medical team.

percutaneous endoscopic gastrostomy (PEG): A procedure whereby a plastic tube is inserted through the abdominal wall and into the stomach for the delivery of nutrition and fluids.

persistent vegetative state: A state of unconsciousness in which a person is kept alive by medical intervention and from which the person has no hope of recovering the ability to think or respond.

Physician Orders for Life-Sustaining Treatment (POLST): A medical care plan signed by a licensed medical doctor for those with advanced illness at any stage; compare MOLST.

platelets: Cells in the bloodstream that help blood to clot, thus stopping bleeding.

pneumonia: An infection in the lungs usually caused by either a bacterium or virus.

prescription drug monitoring program: A computerized system operative in every US state that monitors prescriptions filled for certain high-risk medications, notably narcotics.

red blood cells: Cells that carry oxygen to all parts of the body.

respirator: A mask that filters air to prevent particles from entering a person's airway; compare ventilator.

scheduled drug: A drug classified by the Drug Enforcement Administration as a controlled substance. The DEA classifies certain drugs, chemicals, and other substances according to their presumed risk of abuse, ranging from Schedule 1 (high risk and presumed to have no medical benefit) to Schedule 5 (low risk).

stroke: A condition, with several causes, whereby blood supply to a part of the brain is interrupted.

supportive care: Another term for palliative care that is becoming more commonly used.

terminal condition: A state of health, caused by an injury or illness, from which a person has no hope of recovery and for which curative medical care will only prolong their dying.

utilization review (UR): A cost containment system of evaluation performed by insurance companies and hospitals (and often a source of conflict between the two) for determining whether patients need a longer hospital stay or additional procedures.

ventilator: A machine that provides support for breathing by moving air in and out of the lungs.

white blood cells: Cells that fight infection inside the body.

Resources

AARP (www.aarp.org) has information on many issues facing those over the age of 50, including end-of-life care and advance directives. Advance directive forms for all 50 states and the District of Columbia and Puerto Rico are available from AARP: https://www.aarp.org/caregiving/financial-legal/free-printable-advance-directives/

MyDirectives.com: https://www.mydirectives.com/

CAKE: https://www.joincake.com/

Five Wishes: https://fivewishes.org/
A program connected with https://agingwithdignity.org/

Having the Conversation: https://theconversationproject.org/

MOLST/POLST

>   National POLST organization at https://polst.org/

>   Example of a MOLST form at https://marylandmolst.org/pages/molst_form.htm

National Healthcare Decisions Day, a widely recognized day meant to call attention to the importance of advance care planning, occurs on April 16 every year: https://theconversationproject.org/nhdd/

ORGANIZING SUPPORT

Take Them a Meal: https://takethemameal.com/

CaringBridge.org

Helping Hands: https://lotsahelpinghands.com

PALLIATIVE CARE

Get Palliative Care: www.getpalliativecare.org

HOSPICE CARE

National Hospice and Palliative Care Organization: www.nhpco.org

Hospice Foundation of America: www.hospicefoundation.org

Medicare (https://www.medicare.gov/hospicecompare/): This site lets you compare hospice services.

ORGAN DONATION

Two helpful resources provide complete information and answer frequently asked questions (FAQs) about all aspects of organ donation.

Organ Donor (www.organdonor.gov) is a website managed by the US Department of Health and Human Services. It points out that "each organ and tissue donor saves or improves the lives of as many as 50 people. Giving the 'Gift of Life' may lighten the grief of the donor's own family. Many donor families say that knowing other lives have been saved helps them cope with their tragic loss."

Donate Life America (www.donatelife.net) comprises national organizations and 47 local affiliates across the United States that coordinate donation-related activities at the grassroots level.

ALTERNATIVE FUNERAL AND BURIAL RESOURCES

Funeral Consumers Alliance (www.funerals.org) is a nonprofit organization dedicated to protecting a consumer's right to choose a meaningful, dignified, and affordable funeral. It provides information about funeral options and serves as a consumer advocate for legal and regulatory reform.

HOME FUNERALS

The National Home Funeral Alliance (www.homefuneralalliance.org) supports home funerals and wakes.

NATURAL BURIAL

Natural burial organizations promote burials that are ecologically friendly and less expensive than conventional American funerals. The best national source is the Green Burial Council (www.green burialcouncil.org). There are also state and municipal organizations for natural, or green, burial; look for one where you live.

Ramsey Creek Preserve (http://memorialecosystems.com/) was the first natural burial cemetery in the United States.

BODY DONATION

Body donations can contribute to medical education and research. Donation also avoids funeral and burial expenses. Each state has its own anatomical board that operates body donation programs. Almost all of these boards are affiliated with a university or medical school. A complete listing can be found here: www.med.ufl.edu/anatbd/usprograms.html

Other resources on body donation:

www.anatomicgift.com

www.sciencecare.com

www.biogift.org

PSILOCYBIN AND PSYCHEDELICS

How to Change Your Mind, a book by Michael Pollan

Research by Dr. Roland Griffiths, a Johns Hopkins University professor: https://www.hopkinsmedicine.org

BOOKS

The 36-Hour Day: A Family Guide to Caring for People Who Have Alzheimer Disease, Other Dementias, and Memory Loss, by Nancy L. Mace and Peter V. Rabins, is an excellent resource about dementia.

The Caregiver's Encyclopedia: A Compassionate Guide to Caring for Older Adults, by Muriel R. Gillick, guides people who are taking care of the elderly.

TED TALK ON COMPASSIONOMICS

A 15-minute video recording of Stephen Trzeciak explaining compassionomics to a live audience: www.ted.com/talks/stephen _trzeciak_how_40_seconds_of_compassion_could_save_a_life

MUSIC

There's music from every culture and genre that brings people comfort during difficult times. Here are some of my favorites:

"For a Dancer" by Jackson Browne

"Within You Without You" by The Beatles

"Breathe" by The Kennedys

"When You Walk On" by Eliza Gilkyson

"After All" by Garnet Rogers

Index